DATE DUE FOR RETURN

This book may be recalled before the above date.

MCQs in Pharmacy Practice

Edited by

Lilian M Azzopardi

BPharm, MPhil, PhD

Lecturer
Department of Pharmacy
University of Malta
Msida, Malta

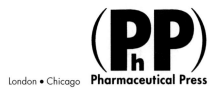

London • Chicago **Pharmaceutical Press**

Published by the Pharmaceutical Press
Publications division of the Royal Pharmaceutical Society of Great Britain

1 Lambeth High Street, London SE1 7JN, UK
100 South Atkinson Road, Suite 206, Grayslake, IL 60030–7820, USA

© Pharmaceutical Press 2004

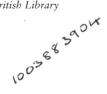 (**PₕP**) is a trade mark of Pharmaceutical Press

First published 2003

Text design by Barker/Hilsdon, Lyme Regis, Dorset
Typeset by Mathematical Composition Setters Ltd, Salisbury, Wiltshire
Printed in Great Britain by TJ International, Padstow, Cornwall

ISBN 0 85369 566 0

A catalogue record for this book is available from the British Library

Contents

Foreword

To practise pharmacy effectively and accountably, it is critical for practitioners to have a sound, contemporary and comprehensive database. In addition to the many good references in textbooks and the periodical literature, there is a certain amount of knowledge that we have to keep current in our memory and daily dialogue. An appropriate balance must be struck by our reliance on memory and our capacity to find, analyse and apply useful knowledge to effective clinical decision making.

Much discussion is currently ongoing around the world of the ideas captured in the phrase 'continuing professional development' (CPD). Simply put, CPD reflects the fact that, for pharmacy professionals to practise with responsibility and accountability, each one must structure a plan and implement mechanisms by which they can maintain their individual competence. It also indicates a willingness of the individual practitioner to build a portfolio of formal and informal educational processes in which they are continuously engaged to ensure competence. They are also willing to have this portfolio reviewed by their peers and perhaps, regulatory bodies, to establish a formal recognition of competence by external parties. Our profession will be examining these precepts over the coming years as a necessary evolution of our thinking around continuing education, public accountability and personal professional development.

Engaging in review of important developments in the field of pharmacy and the disciplines that support its knowledge system is a personal responsibility that all practitioners must take seriously. This is particularly true at this time in the evolution of our profession. As we globally embrace the precepts of pharmaceutical care, as we find an appropriate balance between knowing our products, our patients and their disease states, it is increasingly critical to constantly review new findings as well as legacy principles. One way of doing that is self-assessment.

Shaping a personal way of assessing one's knowledge is an important commitment to continuous professional development and demonstration of personal competence. Self-assessment that is taken seriously has the capacity to identify areas where further 'sharpening' is needed. It also provides the capacity to validate what one knows related to the competence requirements of one's practice. Such assessment is not a comparison of what one knows compared with others but rather, focuses on the skills, knowledge and attitudes that are relevant to an individual's practice.

MCQs in Pharmacy Practice is an important effort to engage individual pharmacists in such self-assessment. The authors of this text have identified a way by which individual pharmacists, who are committed to their own continuing professional development, can apply a systematic way of involving themselves in self assessment. This text provides a guided way of asking important questions, pointing out salient features of rational drug therapy and stimulating deeper thinking through a variety of exercises. Pharmacists who work their way through this book will assuredly gain in their knowledge and skills. More importantly, they will be able to identify those areas in which they may need deeper study.

But going through only this text will not ensure practice competence. The need to stay current with the contemporary literature, involving oneself in formal lecture programmes, being part of intra- and inter-professional scientific dialogue and myriad other ways in which one sharpens one's skills, will still be important engagements. By blending these efforts with structured self-assessment, such as that offered by *MCQs in Pharmacy Practice*, the individual practitioner will have taken major steps in ensuring individual competence.

Henri R Manasse, Jr, BS, MA, PhD, ScD, RPh
Executive Vice President and Chief Executive Officer
American Society of Health-System Pharmacists,
Bethesda, Maryland, USA

Preface

For many years pharmacy education was based on the study of a number of 'classic' basic and applied sciences such as chemistry, mathematics, pharmaceutics, pharmacognosy and pharmacology. Students were then examined separately in these different disciplines. It is only fairly recently that pharmacy practice and pharmaceutical care have been introduced as integral parts of the pharmacy curriculum. Attempts at finding the best way to test the competence of pharmacy students were made at roughly the same time.

Educationalists in many different disciplines have sought ways of testing objectively a student's knowledge of a subject. A perfectly fair examination is one in which students are objectively and accurately assessed with regard to their comprehension, analysis, evaluation and application of all the material with which they have been presented during their course of studies. Multiple choice questions have been accepted as such an objective measure in most areas, including those related to professional practice.

Pharmacy practice has, until very recently, been examined through the traditional essay type of question. This has led, at times, to the feeling that the overall assessment of this discipline could be a subjective one. The MCQ system tries to eliminate the subjective element in an examination and is now well established as a fair mode of assessment. The availability of a pharmacy practice text based on the MCQ system now provides pharmacy students with the opportunity of assessing themselves in the discipline and finding out whether they have mastered it. Dr Azzopardi and her collaborators are to be congratulated in having managed to produce this text. Dr Azzopardi's book has both breadth and depth and should test a student's knowledge rigorously. It should be a welcome addition to the standard texts students use during the years spent in training to become pharmacists.

Roger Ellul-Micallef
Rector, Professor and Head of Department
Clinical Pharmacology and Therapeutics,
University of Malta, Malta

Acknowledgements

I would like to thank my colleagues from the University of Malta, Anthony Serracino-Inglott and Maurice Zarb Adami, who have contributed towards this work, for their ideas and vision. I am also particularly indebted to Sam Salek, University of Cardiff and Steve Hudson, University of Strathclyde for their contributions to this book and for their unflagging cooperation.

Gratitude is also due to Roger Ellul-Micallef, Rector, Godfrey Lafevla, Dean and Mark Brincat, immediate past Dean of the Faculty of Medicine and Surgery, University of Malta for their constant support and guidance. I would like to show my appreciation of Henri J Manasse, Executive Director of the American Society of Health-System Pharmacists, for his interest in the work.

It is proper for me to acknowledge the pharmacy students at the Department of Pharmacy of the University of Malta for their enthusiasm for pharmacy education and for giving us feedback on our efforts.

Thanks also go to the staff of Pharmaceutical Press, particularly Lorraine Parry, and to the staff of the University of Malta, especially Charmaine Borg, for their commitment, work and assistance.

Finally, I would like to thank my sister Louise, a pharmacist who has recently taken preregistration examinations, for her invaluable suggestions and contributions to the book.

About the editor

Lilian M Azzopardi studied pharmacy at the University of Malta, Faculty of Medicine and Surgery. Her inclination to teach shortly led to her appointment in 1994 as a teaching and research assistant. Dr Azzopardi completed an MPhil on the development of formulary systems for community pharmacy in 1995 and in 1999 she gained her PhD, which led to the publication of the book *Validation Instruments for Community Pharmacy: Pharmaceutical Care for the Third Millennium* published in 2000 by Pharmaceutical Products Press, USA. She worked with Professor Anthony Serracino Inglott, who was a pioneer in the introduction of clinical pharmacy in the late sixties.

Dr Azzopardi is currently a lecturer in pharmacy practice at the Department of Pharmacy, University of Malta and is responsible for coordinating the pharmacy practice teaching including the planning, organisation and assessment of pharmacy practice during the undergraduate course as well as in the preregistration period. Dr Azzopardi has examined in pharmacy practice with Professors Anthony Serracino Inglott and Steve Hudson, Dr Sam Salek and Dr Maurice Zarb Adami.

Dr Azzopardi was appointed by the Minister of Health to the Pharmacy Board, which holds the register of pharmacists in Malta. She was for a short period interim director of the European Society of Clinical Pharmacy (ESCP) and is currently coordinator of the ESCP newsletter. She is a member of the Working Group on Quality Care Standards within the Community Pharmacy Section of the International Pharmaceutical Federation (FIP). In 1997 she received an award from the FIP Foundation for Education and Research and in 1999 she was awarded the ESCP German Research and Education Foundation grant.

Lilian Azzopardi has published several papers on clinical pharmacy and pharmaceutical care and has actively participated at congresses organised by FIP, ESCP, the Royal Pharmaceutical Society of Great Britain, the American Pharmaceutical Association and the American Society of Health-System Pharmacists. In 2002 she was invited to contribute to the first sessions of compulsory continuing professional development programme for pharmacists in Italy.

Contributors

Lilian M Azzopardi BPharm, MPhil, PhD
Lecturer, Department of Pharmacy, University of Malta, Msida, Malta

Stephen A Hudson MPharm, MRPharmS
Professor of Pharmaceutical Care, Department of Pharmaceutical Sciences, University of Strathclyde, Glasgow, UK

Sam Salek BPharm, PhD, MRPharmS
Director, Centre for Socioeconomic Research, Welsh School of Pharmacy, Cardiff University, Cardiff, UK

Anthony Serracino-Inglott BPharm, PharmD
Professor and Head of Department, Department of Pharmacy, University of Malta, Msida, Malta

Maurice Zarb-Adami BPharm, PhD
Senior Lecturer, Department of Pharmacy, University of Malta, Msida, Malta

How to use

This book provides an ideal revision guide for those preparing to sit for a multiple choice questions (MCQs) examination in pharmacy. It covers common general pharmacy practice interventions and operations and other topics commonly featured in examinations, such as simple pharmaceutical calculations, doses, strengths, nomenclature, abbreviations, dosage forms, specialities, trade and generic names, biochemical tests, classification, side-effects, and common diseases. Some recent advances in pharmacy practice are also included.

It is recommended that students use this book in their final preparatory stage before sitting for qualifying, licensing or registration examinations so that they are aware of the nature of the questions likely to be posed and how best to approach the examination. This series of MCQ tests is aimed at preparing candidates for their registration examination, whether this is carried out by the state board, the pharmaceutical society or the university. In setting out a broad range of typical MCQs, the aim is to test the level of the candidate's knowledge, as well as helping to reinforce specific points and refine the examination technique.

This book consists of 600 examination-type MCQs. The questions are practice oriented and are intended to assess knowledge, evaluative and analytical skills, and ability to apply that knowledge in clinical practice.

The book consists of two parts. The first is an open-book section wherein the questions aim to assess the student's ability to apply their knowledge in a practice setting in conjunction with the use of information sources. In the second part, the closed-book section, MCQs are directed towards basic skills and knowledge with which the student is expected to be fully familiar.

Each test consists of 100 questions which should be completed in three hours. In each test, different formats of MCQs are adopted. Each format is introduced with directions for answering the MCQs. In each test, case-based and free-standing questions are included. Answers with brief explanations are given at the end of each test.

For each test, write the number of the question and your answer on a separate sheet of paper, then after going through all the questions in the test, compare your answers with those in the book. Attempt one open-book test and one closed-book test so as to mimic examination conditions. Refer to Appendix D for feedback on those questions you did not answer correctly. Information on the proprietary names listed in the book is given in Appendix A. Appendix B includes definitions of medical terms included in the book, while Appendix C lists abbreviations and acronyms.

The recommended textbooks for the open-book section are:

Azzopardi LM (2000). *Validation Instruments for Community Pharmacy: Pharmaceutical Care for the Third Millennium.* Binghamton, New York: Pharmaceutical Products Press.

Edwards C, Stillman P (2000). *Minor illness or Major Disease? Responding to Symptoms in the Pharmacy,* 3rd edn. London: Pharmaceutical Press.

Harman RJ, Mason P, eds (2002). *Handbook of Pharmacy Healthcare: Diseases and Patient Advice,* 2nd edn. London: Pharmaceutical Press.

Mehta DK, ed (2002). *British National Formulary,* 44th edn. London: Pharmaceutical Press.

Nathan A (2002). *Non-prescription Medicines,* 2nd edn. London: Pharmaceutical Press.

Medicines, Ethics and Practice: a Guide for Pharmacists, 26 July 2002. London: Royal Pharmaceutical Society of Great Britain, 2002.

This book is mainly meant for those sitting the final test before being registered as pharmacists. This test is considered to be one of the most challenging tasks in a student's training. The syllabus and specific requirements regarding eligibility to sit for the examination have been carefully laid down by the relevant authorities but the aim is always the same: namely, an attempt to set the required standards of professional skill and ability. The format of the examination itself has been selected to test these standards thoroughly. These preregistration examinations are a necessary obstacle to overcome in becoming a professional pharmacist, in whose hands patients are safe and who is a credit to the profession.

The MCQs method of assessing students is here to stay. MCQs are no longer regarded as an examination that constitutes a final handshake for those who have completed four years at university, passed all the tests, practised in the pharmacy service, gained experience and have received a good report from their mentor pharmacist. Indeed, a poor performance in this assessment may result in overall failure.

MCQs in pharmacy practice do not simply examine facts. Some students expect MCQs to test only factual knowledge. However, questions are also set to test the candidate's ability to comprehend the statements, analyse them and give a logical answer. Some MCQs also test the ability to make safe clinical decisions, and occasionally even test the candidate's professional bearing.

Thorough preparation for an MCQs examination is essential – the information gained and stored during pharmacy practice sessions carried out in a pharmaceutical environment will form the foundation of the candidates' knowledge to enable them to pass the examination.

Preparing and sitting for MCQs in pharmacy practice

Advice about answering MCQs is not very different from that for any other examination, whether oral or written. Starting with dress, there is a tendency to match your psychological outlook and actions to the way you are dressed. Some students approach MCQ tests casually, as if this type of examination were not as serious an undertaking as any other. Have a shower beforehand and men, have a clean shave, as these all help you to concentrate. Dress smartly but comfortably and conservatively. Avoid clothes that make you feel too relaxed, such as casual jackets or leisure wear. Women should avoid extremely short skirts or low necklines, which might distract from the task in hand. Arrive a little early for the examination and plan how much time to allocate for each question, allowing extra time for more difficult questions.

Open-book examinations

The rarity of absolutes in pharmacy practice means that a variety of adjectives and adverbs are commonly used in its description, increasing the difficulty of answering MCQs. Although the desirability of assessing knowledge that is dependent on the 'strength' of an adjective can be questioned, these adjectives do form part of the language of present-day pharmacy practice, borne out by their frequent use in the questions and answers presented in this book. You should not assume they are clues – they may or may not be.

The following are suggestions about how to tackle the questions in Test 1 of this book. These pointers may be applied to the other tests in this publication. The questions are tackled in groups and a number of points are considered. However, some of the points discussed may certainly be adopted in answering other questions. Sometimes the open-book questions may even present more of a challenge than the closed-book questions. In the case of Test 1, which is an open-book examination, there is also advice about the best use of reference books within the time allowed for answering the MCQs.

Questions 1–25

Several questions contain the statement: 'All ... EXCEPT'. In this book, 'except' is in capital letters (upper case) but not all texts use this convention. More important is the fact that only *one* answer – *one* choice – is allowed. This is explained in the statement at the beginning of the questions.

Never underestimate the importance of reading the directions very carefully. In this case, the directions state: 'Select the best answer in each case.' (Note the use of the word 'best'.) Do not spend too much time, however, selecting the 'best' answer – very often there is only one *correct* answer. Candidates who select more than one answer will not be given any marks, even if the choice includes the correct answer.

Another type of question includes the word 'NOT' – again this book uses upper case but this may not be so in all examinations, so watch out for such words (for example, in Q4).

Do not be unduly perturbed by the word 'appropriate' when it is stated that there is only one correct answer. The chances are that there is only one 'therapeutic alternative' (Q6). 'Appropriate' is used only as a linguistic necessity because, if it were omitted, then the other alternatives might be possible, if not appropriate. In practice, however, no other 'alternative' is available except the correct answer. 'Appropriate' is therefore superfluous and should not bother you. Focus more on the term 'bed-ridden', which is an indication of possible long-term use of the laxative (Q8).

The same applies to 'optimum' in Q12. There is only one correct range for plasma theophylline concentrations. 'Optimum' here is again a nicety of the language.

Be careful about the use of 'over-the-counter', which actually means 'without a prescription'. Note that the emphasis is rarely on 'over-the-counter' but on the condition. In Q13 the term is again superfluous and you should not be confused by it. 'Over-the-counter' is often introduced to denote that this is a pharmacy practice examination and therefore the exceptional use of substances indicated only in very rare cases is excluded.

Similarly, 'because' means a description of an action of a drug and so, in questions such as Q14, the importance of the drug rather than the disease should be stressed. However, if you do not know the action of the specific drug then a good suggestion would be to look at the disease and examine what action is required to address the particular ailment.

Other terms are used, such as 'differs', which does not necessarily mean 'different from'; in Q20 the question refers to a *total* difference in the components of the products. 'Equivalent to' usually means having the same active ingredients, or a drug belonging to the same class, and not equivalent in 'use' or in 'action' (Q23).

MCQs, contrary to what some students fear, are not meant to be tricky. Do not try to read between the lines but do read the statements very carefully. Many mistakes happen because the directions are not carefully followed. This kind of exercise is part of the test itself, as in pharmacy practice, mistakes are often made because a prescription or the patient's drug profile have not been properly read.

Questions 26–52

The tests are set so that there are 100 questions with an open-book option, and another 100 questions of the closed-book type. Questions in both formats may appear to be complex in their setting. Devote enough time to understand the question clearly. Statements or advice that a heading may be used once, more than once or not at all mean exactly that.

The term 'most closely related to' (*see* directions for Q26–52) is not a 'trick' and you should not expect to find some statements more closely related than others. Very often only one statement is obviously related and it is safe to assume that the other answers are incorrect. Do not be misled by the use of 'most closely', which is actually superfluous.

In an open-book situation, expect a number of proprietary (trade) names or diseases. Although candidates are allowed to look up all the trade names in the textbooks available, in an examination this is not practical and sometimes impossible to achieve in the allocated time. Check the active ingredients of a proprietary name only when necessary or when in doubt. You are expected to have a good knowledge of most brands and pharmaceutical manufacturers (Q26–40).

Diseases tend to present a distinct challenge to pharmacy practice examination candidates. Students often do their best to gain as much knowledge of drugs as possible, but when it comes to diseases they are confused. There are so many thousands of diseases, where should one start? Which diseases should be revised for an MCQs examination? What depth of knowledge about diseases is expected? In tackling these questions it is important to be very familiar with the textbooks used in the open-book examination. Very often the rule of thumb is 'the simpler, the better', so do *not* take encyclopaedias with you to the examination. A book such as *Martindale: the Complete Drug Reference* may be useful but it is not essential and would only be used on a few occasions. However, a reference such as the *British National Formulary* (BNF) should be kept at hand. For this book, the 44th edition (September 2002) was used.

Let us examine how, for example, Q32–34 could be tackled by the following steps:

1   Write the generic names next to A–E, starting with those that you are confident about.
2   Find the ones you do not know, or are unsure of, in the BNF index (at this stage, just note the page numbers).
3   Find the generic names by going through the pages, checking the list in alphabetical order, rather than going backwards and forwards, to save time.

(Any reference books to be used in the examination should not be bought at the last moment – books should have been used for some time because it is easier to turn the pages, as those in new books tend to stick together; such minor annoyances encountered during an examination can increase the tension. In addition, get used to the newer editions of the textbooks. Practise using the indexes, appendices and footnotes and be familiar with the overall structure of the reference books used in an open-book session.)

The phrase 'associated with' used, for example, in Q35–37, means only 'who is the manufacturer of that particular drug?' This information should not be sought, say, in a pharmacology text-book but can be easily located in a formulary such as the BNF. First write the page numbers next to Q35–37, after finding them in the index (preferably in alphabetical order to save time) and then find the corresponding pages in the text. You will find the manufacturer's name in parentheses next to the product name.

Although in Q32–34 you only had to look for the products A–E and match them with the specific diseases, in Q35–37, do not attempt to find the manufacturers A–E; look up the three products instead. Q38–40 should be attempted in the same way as Q32–34.

Practise these simple techniques, although they seem obvious when you know about them, as this type of question can cause confusion when met unawares and could be a challenge even to the diligent student who studied the facts but who had no practice with MCQs.

The next group of questions refers more to diseases and bio-chemical tests (Q41–44). These questions present more of a problem, not because of their difficulty but owing to the technique needed to make the best use of the reference books available. In this case follow these steps:

1   Write the page numbers next to the choices A–E after con-sulting a drug index or formulary that you know carries pre-cautions to be taken with the use of drugs, e.g. the BNF.

2   Write in summary format the biochemical test/disease men-tioned in these questions, namely: (Q41) liver function tests; (Q42) epilepsy; (Q43) thyroid function; (Q44) peptic ulcer.

3   In the BNF, look under cautions for levodopa – the second one listed is peptic ulceration, so put A next to Q44. For domperidone, there are only three lines of cautions, none listing any of the four conditions, so go straight on to con-sider fluvastatin. (When consulting the index, always note down and look up the page marked in bold first.) Under cau-tions for all statins, in the first few lines there is a statement

advising a liver function test. In an examination, if you are pressed for time, do not continue reading all the cautions but move on immediately to the next drug after marking C next to Q41.

A good reminder is that a reference book in an open-book examination should be used just to support your knowledge and only in rare cases to find unknown data. The availability of books in an examination does not replace the need for studying, particularly basic facts that require instant recall. Lack of this kind of preparation is often one of the reasons why some candidates perform worse in an open-book examination than in a closed-book one. Do not expect to gather all the information during the examination – the questions are designed to ensure that only students who are well versed and properly trained in pharmacy practice will pass.

Questions 53–83

These questions (Q53–83), which present a choice of answers grouped together, are a common format that sometimes perplexes students. The system is not meant to confuse but is used to facilitate the marking procedure. In this book the directions are summarised in a box but this may not always be the case in examinations set by different boards. Follow these steps to answer this type of question:

1 Summarise the directions if not already presented this way.
2 Mark the correct statements as if they were true/false answers.
3 Collate the answers.
4 Match the collated answers with the letters A–E, as indicated in the directions.
5 Write your chosen letter next to the question.

Do not answer the questions by writing '1, 2' or '1, 2, 3' or 'T' or 'F' but follow the instructions exactly and put a letter A–E. The reverse is also true, that is, if you are asked to write numbers (in a rare case) or T and F, do not create your own summary. Remember that answer papers are sometimes corrected by clerks, who are given strict rules for recording correct answers, which they are obliged to follow. More commonly today, the analysis is undertaken by computer, so not following the instructions may result in the answer being marked as incorrect, no matter what was written. In Test 1 in this book, for example, Q53–83, i.e. 30% of the examination, are given in this format. There have been reports that some students lost 30% of their marks simply because they did not follow the instructions.

It must be emphasised that, although all the information required to answer the questions correctly is available in the recommended textbooks, do not try to verify all the information. In Q58, for example, you need to read the question carefully – in this case, the emphasis is on the word 'daily'. The information can be found in the BNF under 'monitoring' but it is time consuming to read it all very carefully and, in this type of question, it is better to spend more time carefully examining the statements, rather than browsing through the books. This is totally different from using the book to check a dosage regimen, a proprietary name or a caution.

Similarly in Q55 the word 'care' should not be confused with a contraindication. The BNF states under cautions: 'Reduce dose in the elderly'. This should be interpreted that care should be taken with the use of digoxin. You may ask – should care not be taken with the use of *all* medicines, especially in the elderly? In this context, the word 'care' should be taken as meaning with *special* care or caution.

Questions 58–63 refer to diseases. In addition to using formularies such as the BNF, in this case, you may need to refer to other textbooks such as *Minor Illness or Major Disease* (*see* Bibliography) to answer these types of questions. In tackling Q61, the emphasis that the textbook places on detection combing for head lice signifies that this is the diagnostic process. This indicates how important it is that an authorative book is used in an examination when you are allowed a choice of textbooks. The use of such books will help you find the correct answer, even when the answer is not specifically stated as such but needs to be inferred. The textbook selected for use in open-book MCQs should have an extensive index for quick reference.

In Q63, dealing with tinea pedis, a glance at the index of a good textbook will immediately remind you that this is athlete's foot. Many textbooks give a summary but sometimes it is worth going beyond this. The whole text on the topic itself is, in some cases, only a short paragraph. In dealing with Q63, for example, if you restrict yourself to the summary, you may miss the fact that the maceration is white, as the description of the earlier stage of tinea pedis is described in the summary as a 'red eruption' in *Minor Illness or Major Disease*.

Questions 64–71 concern drug use, contraindications, cautions and side-effects, which may all be found in formularies such as the BNF. It is important to look under the drug names rather than try to find information by looking for a disease or symptom.

Some questions may take the form of a case study (Q72). These should be analysed as if the patient were presenting at the pharmacy. In this case, start with the diagnosis – here it is clearly a case of verruca. Once this step has been taken, the correct diagnosis can be confirmed by quick reference to a note on verrucas given, for example, in *Minor Illness or Major Disease*.

Another textbook recommended for use in questions that concern conditions rather than medicines is *Handbook of Pharmacy Healthcare: Diseases and Patient Advice* (*see* Bibliography). The book could be useful to answer questions such as 73–74 and 82–83.

Questions 84–88

Questions 84–88 appear to be more complex than the rest. The choices C, D or E are simple true or false answers to the statements. The choice between A and B, however, depends on whether the second statement is an explanation of the first statement. In this book, the questions in this section carry clear directions and even a summary to help you understand how to tackle them. This may not be the case in all board examinations, so practise how to summarise complex directions.

The aim of the questions is to test your ability to reach logical conclusions. The correctness of the statements can be verified in the textbooks but the logic of the sequence cannot. This type of question is becoming more popular with examiners because it tests an important aspect of pharmacy practice, namely logical argument from data that can be extracted from books but which then has to be interpreted in the practical setting.

Questions 89–100

The dispensing of prescriptions is considered to be a primary function in pharmacy practice. This is tackled in the final part of the test (Q89–94). The statements on Xenical can all be found in the BNF, except for the one stating that it 'may be administered twice daily'. The answer to this part is in the prescription presented (bd) in the question itself. This instance is a clear example pointing to the need to read the prescription carefully (Q89–90).

In the case of the prescription relating to Daktacort (Q91–94), for candidates not familiar with its use, it is important to identify the active ingredients. Daktacort is listed in the BNF under hydrocortisone but its main use is as an antifungal agent. The need to apply the cream sparingly results from the steroid content and its use twice rather than three times daily comes from the information on the prescription (bd).

Some proprietary names may not be familiar to certain candidates, because an effort has been made to make this book suitable for different countries. If you do not recognise the brand name, use Appendix A, where the active ingredients of all proprietary products listed in the book are included. Irfen, for example (Q96), is not listed in the BNF but you can find information about it in Appendix A.

Finally, to conclude these pointers on the open-book questions, let us look at the statistics for Test 1 presented in Appendix D. These statistics were recorded following the tests carried out by a sample of final-year students after a five-year university course which included the preregistration period. In Test 1, the questions that were answered incorrectly by the highest number of students were 58, 61, 62 and 86, whereas the ones most often answered correctly were 1, 14, 15, 17, 22, 25, 26, 30, 33, 41, 52, 67, 81, 89, 91 and 98. Questions answered incorrectly were often those that required some logical thinking. A good lesson to conclude this section, therefore, is that no textbook should replace logical thinking, even during an open-book examination.

Closed-book examinations

Most of the advice given for the open-book examinations should also be kept in mind for the closed-book tests. It is essential to revise the major classes of drugs, comparing the use, unwanted effects, contraindications and alternative products available. In this section, Test 4 is used as the example to highlight the following areas for quick revision:

- cautionary labels (Q2)
- adverse effects (Q4, Q27)
- calculations (Q6, Q11, Q17, Q18)
- contraindications (Q7)
- drug interactions (Q8)
- pregnancy (Q9, Q80)
- extemporaneous preparations (Q3)
- disease management and drug indications (Q1, Q14, Q38; *see* Appendix B for short descriptions of diseases)
- drug classification (Q12, Q16, Q22, Q56)
- proprietary names (Q13, Q28; *see* Appendix A)
- aetiology of disease (Q19)
- drug indications (Q25, Q26, Q29)

- drug actions (Q24, Q45–48)
- drug formulation (Q34, Q49)
- abbreviations (Q42–44; *see* Appendix C)
- disease symptoms (Q39–41, Q53; *see* Appendix B)
- predisposing factors and risk factors (Q54, Q65)
- prophylaxis (Q57)
- pharmacist interventions (Q75).

A good look at the index of this book indicates the items commonly encountered in examinations. The index is an exhaustive one and is divided into proprietary names, generic names, subject areas and conditions. A self-assessment exercise is to check that you have adequate knowledge of examples of the topics listed above and then attempt the tests. A review of the drugs in the index provides examples of medicines that certainly need attention. You should be familiar with the action, classification, side-effects, clinically significant drug interactions, contraindications and cautions of a number of classes of drugs, such as:

- antibacterials (e.g. penicillins, cephalosporins, ciprofloxacin, metronidazole, doxycycline)
- analgesics (e.g. codeine, tramadol, co-proxamol, paracetamol, non-steroidal anti-inflammatory drugs)
- vitamins and minerals (e.g. iron, folic acid, vitamin A, C, E, B_{12})
- cardiovascular drugs (e.g. thiazide diuretics, digoxin, beta-adrenoceptor blocking drugs, calcium-channel blockers, drugs acting on the renin–angiotensin system)
- antidiabetic (e.g. glibenclamide, gliclazide, metformin, insulin)
- gastrointestinal drugs (e.g. antacids, proton pump inhibitors, laxatives)
- anti-asthmatic therapy (e.g. bronchodilators, corticosteroids)

Using the index it is possible to gain an insight into the selection of drugs covered in such examinations. Check that you know the meaning of the conditions listed in Appendix B and make lists of medicines that are indicated and contraindicated or that may precipitate the condition.

Finally, examining the statistics for Test 4 regarding questions that were answered incorrectly by the largest number of candidates, it can be concluded that nothing can replace practical observation during the in-service training in a pharmacy, for example, knowledge of the expiration date of extemporaneous preparations is information that is acquired during practice sessions (Q3). The use of medicines for prophylaxis, rather than for treatment, is often confused by candidates, as can be seen from the statistics for Q59, where allopurinol was mistaken for *treatment* of gout when it is indicated for *prophylactic* use. Some questions require reasoning rather than just recall of information, such as Q80 and Q93. Practise reasoning out answers when undertaking self-assessment questions before the examination.

Questions 8, 17, 20, 26, 39, 46, 49, 51, 70 and 88 were answered incorrectly by less than 5% of the candidates. It is advisable to tackle these questions first, as they ought to be answered easily, allowing more time for the questions where reasoning is required. Appendix D indicates which questions were the hardest. This should serve as a guide and can give feedback on how you would compare with colleagues in a qualifying or licensing and registration examination.

Note

Use of Names for Medicinal Substances

The recommended International Non-proprietary Name (rINN) is used throughout the book, except when the terms used are adrenaline and noradrenaline with any former UK names in parentheses. For further reference, see the *British National Formulary*.

Dosage Forms

In the answers to questions and in Appendix A, when no mention of a dosage form (e.g. tablets, lotion, drops) is made, the data refer to the dosage form indicated in the questions.

Section 1

Open-book Questions

Test 1

Questions

Questions 1–25

Directions: Each of the questions or incomplete statements is followed by five suggested answers. Select the best answer in each case.

Q1   All of the following products contain hydrocortisone EXCEPT:

A   ☐ Fucidin H
B   ☐ Daktacort
C   ☐ Fucicort
D   ☐ Hydrocortisyl
E   ☐ Canesten HC

Q2   All of the following accompanying symptoms for headache warrant referral EXCEPT:

A   ☐ loss of consciousness
B   ☐ neck stiffness
C   ☐ paraesthesia
D   ☐ slurred speech
E   ☐ fever

Q3   Nifedipine:

A   ☐ constricts vascular smooth muscle
B   ☐ long-acting formulations are preferred in the long-term treatment of hypertension

C ☐ is a nitrate

D ☐ interferes with the inward displacement of potassium ions through active cell membranes

E ☐ results in increased risk of bradycardia when administered concomitantly with atenolol

Q4 Which of the following is NOT involved in the presentation of seasonal allergic rhinitis?

A ☐ leukotrienes

B ☐ prostaglandins

C ☐ osteocytes

D ☐ basophils

E ☐ mast cells

Q5 Patient medication records should include all EXCEPT:

A ☐ medication allergies

B ☐ diagnosis

C ☐ current medication therapy

D ☐ pets kept at home

E ☐ age

Q6 What is an appropriate therapeutic alternative for Uniflu?

A ☐ Actifed

B ☐ Day Nurse

C ☐ Phenergan

D ☐ Ventolin

E ☐ Xyzal

Q7   Symptoms of vaginal candidiasis that warrant referral include all EXCEPT:

A   ☐ vaginal discharge

B   ☐ abdominal pain

C   ☐ fever

D   ☐ diabetes

E   ☐ pregnancy

Q8   An appropriate laxative preparation for an elderly patient who is bed-ridden is:

A   ☐ bisacodyl

B   ☐ senna

C   ☐ magnesium sulphate

D   ☐ lactulose

E   ☐ liquid paraffin

Q9   All of the following drugs affect the renin–angiotensin system EXCEPT:

A   ☐ hydralazine

B   ☐ valsartan

C   ☐ losartan

D   ☐ perindopril

E   ☐ enalapril

Q10   A significant clinical interaction may occur if lithium is administered concomitantly with:

A   ☐ paroxetine

B   ☐ glibenclamide

C   ☐ co-amoxiclav

D   ☐ atenolol

E   ☐ nifedipine

Q11 Rofecoxib:

A ☐ has a similar effect to diclofenac

B ☐ provides protection against ischaemic cardiovascular events

C ☐ is indicated for long-term use in osteoarthritis

D ☐ is not contraindicated in patients with active peptic ulceration

E ☐ is marketed under the proprietary name Mobic

Q12 For optimum response, plasma theophylline concentration should be maintained at:

A ☐ 30–40 mg/L

B ☐ 2–5 mg/L

C ☐ 8–10 mg/L

D ☐ 10–20 mg/L

E ☐ 20–25 mg/L

Q13 Appropriate preparations which could be dispensed over-the-counter to treat motion sickness include all of the following EXCEPT:

A ☐ Stugeron

B ☐ Avomine

C ☐ Biodramina

D ☐ Motilium

E ☐ Phenergan

Q14 Alfuzosin is used in benign prostatic hyperplasia because it:

A ☐ lowers blood pressure

B ☐ decreases urinary flow rate

C ☐ constricts smooth muscle

D ☐ increases bladder capacity

E ☐ relaxes smooth muscle

Q15   Which of the following antibacterial agents is not presented for systemic use?

A   ☐ sodium fusidate
B   ☐ vancomycin
C   ☐ gentamicin
D   ☐ mupirocin
E   ☐ doxycycline

Q16   All of the following products are Controlled Drugs EXCEPT:

A   ☐ pethidine
B   ☐ diazepam
C   ☐ morphine
D   ☐ alfentanil
E   ☐ phenazocine

Q17   Famciclovir is:

A   ☐ an ester of aciclovir
B   ☐ too toxic for systemic use
C   ☐ a pro-drug of penciclovir
D   ☐ not indicated in acute genital herpes simplex
E   ☐ indicated for the prophylaxis of varicella zoster

Q18   All of the following factors could precipitate the onset of herpes labialis EXCEPT:

A   ☐ common cold
B   ☐ sun
C   ☐ trauma to the lips
D   ☐ dental caries
E   ☐ immunosuppression

Q19   A preparation that is available in eye drops and as an eye ointment is:

A   ☐   Fucithalmic

B   ☐   Soframycin

C   ☐   Zovirax

D   ☐   Livostin

E   ☐   Timoptol

Q20   Cilest differs from Microgynon in that it:

A   ☐   is used in hormone replacement therapy

B   ☐   is available for transdermal drug delivery

C   ☐   has to be taken twice daily

D   ☐   contains norgestimate

E   ☐   can be used in patients with venous thromboembolic disease

Q21   What is the most appropriate treatment that could be dispensed over-the-counter for irritation due to contact dermatitis?

A   ☐   Histergan cream

B   ☐   Travocort cream

C   ☐   Hydrocortisyl cream

D   ☐   Clarityn tablets

E   ☐   Pevaryl sachets

Q22   Which of the following products is NOT indicated for the treatment of insomnia?

A   ☐   Stilnoct

B   ☐   diazepam

C   ☐   Heminevrin

D   ☐   Buspar

E   ☐   Phenergan

Q23 Which of the following products may be recommended as an equivalent to Rhinocort Aqua?

A ☐ Livostin
B ☐ Otrivine
C ☐ Beconase
D ☐ Dexa-Rhinaspray Duo
E ☐ Rhinocap

Q24 Bupivacaine:

A ☐ has a rapid onset of action
B ☐ is suitable for continuous epidural analgesia in labour
C ☐ is of short duration of action
D ☐ is used in dentistry
E ☐ is presented in Xylocaine

Q25 Haloperidol is used in the treatment of all of the following conditions EXCEPT:

A ☐ motor tics
B ☐ schizophrenia
C ☐ intractable hiccup
D ☐ parkinsonism
E ☐ severe anxiety

Questions 26–52

Directions: Each group of questions below consists of five lettered headings followed by a list of numbered questions. For each numbered question select the one heading that is most closely related to it. Each heading may be used once, more than once, or not at all.

Questions 26–28 concern the following vaccines:

A ☐ Twinrix
B ☐ ACT-HIB
C ☐ Engerix B
D ☐ Fluarix
E ☐ Havrix

Select from A to E, which one of the above:

Q26 covers against hepatitis A and B

Q27 is not normally required for children over 4 years

Q28 contains the H and N component of the prevalent strains as indicated by the World Health Organization

Questions 29–31 concern the following products:

A ☐ Zinnat
B ☐ Zofran
C ☐ Cytotec
D ☐ Indocid
E ☐ Diamox

Select from A to E, the product that can cause:

Q29 constipation

Q30 abnormal vaginal bleeding

Q31 paraesthesia

Questions 32–34 concern the following products:

A   ☐   Cardura
B   ☐   Inderal
C   ☐   Cozaar
D   ☐   Tildiem
E   ☐   Aldactone

Select from **A** to **E**, the product that should be used with caution in the following conditions:

Q32   porphyria

Q33   diabetes

Q34   myasthenia gravis

Questions 35–37 concern the following manufacturers:

A   ☐   AstraZeneca
B   ☐   Schering-Plough
C   ☐   Boehringer Ingelheim
D   ☐   Lilly
E   ☐   Abbott

Select from **A** to **E**, which one of the above manufacturers is associated with the trademarked product:

Q35   Nu-Seals

Q36   Bricanyl

Q37   Alupent

Questions 38–40 concern the following products:

A   ☐ Karvol
B   ☐ Livostin
C   ☐ Difflam
D   ☐ Molcer
E   ☐ Daktarin

Select from A to E, the product that is presented in the following dosage forms:

Q38   oral rinse

Q39   nasal spray

Q40   ear drops

Questions 41–44 concern the following drugs:

A   ☐ levodopa
B   ☐ domperidone
C   ☐ fluvastatin
D   ☐ lithium
E   ☐ fluvoxamine

Select from A to E, which of the above:

Q41   should prompt liver function tests before initiating treatment

Q42   should be used with caution in patients with epilepsy

Q43   requires monitoring of thyroid function

Q44   should be used with caution in patients with peptic ulcer disease

Questions 45–48 concern the following strengths:

A   ☐   2 mg
B   ☐   150 mg
C   ☐   5 mg
D   ☐   10 mg
E   ☐   200 mg

Select from **A** to **E**, a strength in which the following products are available:

Q45   Dulcolax tablets

Q46   Zantac tablets

Q47   Phenergan tablets

Q48   Imodium capsules

Questions 49–52 concern the following drugs:

A   ☐   norfloxacin
B   ☐   nabumetone
C   ☐   nifedipine
D   ☐   nalidixic acid
E   ☐   nefazodone

Select from **A** to **E**, which one of the above corresponds to the drug brand name:

Q49   Mictral

Q50   Noroxin

Q51   Relifex

Q52   Adalat

Questions 53–83

Directions: For each of the questions below, ONE or MORE of the responses is (are) correct. Decide which of the responses is (are) correct. Then choose:

A ❑ if 1, 2 and 3 are correct
B ❑ if 1 and 2 only are correct
C ❑ if 2 and 3 only are correct
D ❑ if 1 only is correct
E ❑ if 3 only is correct

Directions summarised				
A	B	C	D	E
1, 2, 3	1, 2 only	2, 3 only	1 only	3 only

Q53   When dispensing acarbose, the patient should be advised:

1 ❑ to take tablets in the morning
2 ❑ to avoid direct sunlight
3 ❑ that flatulence and diarrhoea may occur

Q54   Side-effects of esomeprazole include:

1 ❑ headache
2 ❑ pruritus
3 ❑ dizziness

Q55   Care should be taken with the use of the following drug(s) in older patients:

1 ❑ digoxin
2 ❑ trihexyphenidyl (benzhexol)
3 ❑ lactulose

Q56 When dispensing mefloquine as a prophylaxis against malaria, the patient should be advised that:

1 ☐ prophylaxis has to be taken regularly
2 ☐ mosquito bites should be avoided
3 ☐ dizziness may occur as a side-effect

Q57 Symptoms of venous thrombosis include:

1 ☐ oedema
2 ☐ lower leg becoming bluish in colour
3 ☐ dry skin

Q58 In diabetes, blood glucose monitoring by the patient is of benefit:

1 ☐ to detect hypoglycaemia
2 ☐ to observe fluctuations in blood glucose over 24 h
3 ☐ to make daily adjustments to insulin dose

Q59 Carcinoma of the large bowel could present:

1 ☐ with symptoms of bowel obstruction
2 ☐ at an advanced stage
3 ☐ with melaena

Q60 Clinical signs of tuberculosis include:

1 ☐ persistent cough
2 ☐ fever
3 ☐ weight loss

Q61 Diagnosis of head lice infestation is based on:

1 ☐ detection combing
2 ☐ itchy scalp
3 ☐ hair cleanliness

Q62 Which of the symptoms are characteristic of acute bronchitis?

1 ☐ chest tightness
2 ☐ purulent sputum
3 ☐ wheeziness

Q63 Symptoms of tinea pedis include:

1 ☐ itchiness
2 ☐ location mostly in interdigital space
3 ☐ white, macerated skin

Q64 Interferon beta:

1 ☐ can be administered orally and parenterally
2 ☐ may cause myalgia and fever
3 ☐ is used in multiple sclerosis

Q65 Tamoxifen:

1 ☐ is an oestrogen receptor agonist
2 ☐ presents a risk of endometrial cancer
3 ☐ is used in breast cancer in post-menopausal women with metastatic disease

Q66 Bromocriptine should be used with caution in:

1 ☐ renal impairment
2 ☐ schizophrenia
3 ☐ pregnancy

Q67 Which of the following cytotoxic drugs can be administered orally?

1 ☐ capecitabine
2 ☐ cyclophosphamide
3 ☐ carboplatin

Q68   Dydrogesterone:

1   ☐ is a progesterone analogue
2   ☐ is indicated for endometriosis
3   ☐ is contraindicated in severe liver impairment

Q69   Which of the products could be used to counteract the vasomotor symptoms associated with menopause?

1   ☐ Premarin
2   ☐ Livial
3   ☐ Logynon

Q70   Side-effects associated with testosterone include:

1   ☐ headache
2   ☐ hirsutism
3   ☐ gynaecomastia

Q71   Levofloxacin:

1   ☐ has greater activity against pneumococci than ciprofloxacin
2   ☐ should be used with caution in patients with a history of epilepsy
3   ☐ may cause tremor and tachycardia

Q72   A patient presents at the pharmacy with a lesion, which appears to be a hard plaque with a central black area, on the underside of the foot:

1   ☐ patient should be referred immediately
2   ☐ patient should be asked about medical history of diabetes
3   ☐ products containing salicylic acid can be recommended

Q73   Lichen planus:

1   ☐ may involve gingival tissue
2   ☐ treatment may involve corticosteroids
3   ☐ pruritus occurs in most cases

Q74   Chickenpox:

1   ☐ is caused by herpes simplex
2   ☐ could be contracted from contact with a patient with shingles
3   ☐ promethazine could be used

Q75   Terbinafine:

1   ☐ is the drug of choice in onchomycosis
2   ☐ could cause photosensitivity
3   ☐ treatment should not exceed 2 weeks

Q76   For anti-lice lotions:

1   ☐ alcoholic formulations are more effective
2   ☐ alcoholic formulations should be avoided in asthmatic patients
3   ☐ routine use is recommended as a prophylaxis

Q77   Rosiglitazone:

1   ☐ is a biguanide
2   ☐ should not be used with gliclazide
3   ☐ should be used with caution in patients with cardiovascular disease

Q78   Compared with soluble insulin, insulin aspart:

1   ☐ has a faster onset of action
2   ☐ results in a higher fasting blood–glucose concentration
3   ☐ is associated with a lower frequency of hypoglycaemia

Q79 Fluconazole:

1 ☐ may be used in vaginal candidiasis
2 ☐ is a triazole antifungal
3 ☐ when administered concomitantly with glibenclamide results in a lower plasma concentration of glibenclamide

Q80 Which of the following statements about cradle cap is (are) true?

1 ☐ it is a form of seborrhoeic dermatitis
2 ☐ baby oil could be used to relieve the condition
3 ☐ it is contagious

Q81 Examples of non-steroidal anti-inflammatory products include:

1 ☐ Oruvail
2 ☐ Feldene
3 ☐ Nootropil

Q82 For which of the following infections is antibacterial treatment NOT usually recommended:

1 ☐ typhoid fever
2 ☐ impetigo
3 ☐ gastroenteritis

Q83 The following is (are) effective in the management of nappy rash:

1 ☐ zinc and castor oil ointment
2 ☐ Anthisan cream
3 ☐ Eurax cream

Questions 84–88

Directions: The following questions consist of a first statement followed by a second statement. Decide whether the first statement is true or false. Decide whether the second statement is true or false. Then choose:

A   ❏ if both statements are true and the second statement is a **correct explanation** of the first statement

B   ❏ if both statements are true but the second statement **is NOT a correct explanation** of the first statement

C   ❏ if the first statement is true but the second statement is false

D   ❏ if the first statement is false but the second statement is true

E   ❏ if both statements are false

Directions summarised			
	First statement	**Second statement**	
A	True	True	Second statement is a *correct explanation* of the first
B	True	True	Second statement is *NOT a correct explanation* of the first
C	True	False	
D	False	True	
E	False	False	

Q84   Paclitaxel is a cytotoxic antibiotic. Paclitaxel is used in primary ovarian cancer.

Q85   The combination of antibacterial agents in co-trimoxazole presents a synergistic activity. Co-trimoxazole is associated with rare but serious side-effects.

Q86 Pethidine is a less potent analgesic than morphine. Pethidine is not suitable for severe, continuous pain.

Q87 All tetracyclines are effective against *Neisseria meningitidis*. Tetracyclines are used in acne.

Q88 Zafirlukast is a leukotriene-receptor antagonist. Zafirlukast is used in the treatment of an acute severe asthma attack.

Questions 89–100

Directions: These questions involve cases. Read the prescription or case and answer the questions.

Questions 89–90: Use the prescription below:

Patient's name   ....

Xenical capsules
1 caps b.d. p.c.   m. 30

Doctor's signature   ....

Q89 In which condition is the product used?

A   ☐ anorexia
B   ☐ asthenia
C   ☐ obesity
D   ☐ bulimia
E   ☐ cholestasis

Q90   Xenical

1   ☐   is a pancreatic lipase inhibitor
2   ☐   may cause faecal urgency
3   ☐   may be administered twice daily

A   ☐   1, 2, 3
B   ☐   1, 2 only
C   ☐   2, 3 only
D   ☐   1 only
E   ☐   3 only

Questions 91–94: Use the prescription below:

Patient's name   ....

Daktacort cream
b.d. for 1 week   m. 1 tube

Doctor's signature   ....

Q91   The active ingredient(s) of Daktacort is (are):

A   ☐   econazole
B   ☐   hydrocortisone
C   ☐   econazole, hydrocortisone
D   ☐   miconazole, hydrocortisone
E   ☐   miconazole

Q92   Daktacort

1   ☐ is rarely associated with side-effects
2   ☐ should be discarded 5 days after opening
3   ☐ is also available as powder

A   ☐ 1, 2, 3
B   ☐ 1, 2 only
C   ☐ 2, 3 only
D   ☐ 1 only
E   ☐ 3 only

Q93   Daktacort is prescribed when the patient has:

A   ☐ fungal infection
B   ☐ dry skin
C   ☐ bacterial infection
D   ☐ acne
E   ☐ psoriasis

Q94   The pharmacist should advise the patient to apply Daktacort

1   ☐ sparingly
2   ☐ three times daily
3   ☐ for 6 months

A   ☐ 1, 2, 3
B   ☐ 1, 2 only
C   ☐ 2, 3 only
D   ☐ 1 only
E   ☐ 3 only

Questions 95–100: Use the patient profile below:

Patient medication profile

Patient's name   ....

Age   42 years

Allergies   none

Diagnosis   peptic ulcer disease, hypertension

Prescribed medication   amoxicillin 1 g b.d.
omeprazole 20 mg b.d.
clarithromycin 500 mg b.d.

Q95   The duration of treatment which has been prescribed is usually:

A   ☐ 7 days
B   ☐ 3 days
C   ☐ 30 days
D   ☐ 5 days
E   ☐ 10 days

Q96   The pharmacist should advise the patient against the use of:

1   ☐ Irfen
2   ☐ Clarityn
3   ☐ Rennie

A   ☐ 1, 2, 3
B   ☐ 1, 2 only
C   ☐ 2, 3 only
D   ☐ 1 only
E   ☐ 3 only

Q97   Adverse effects that could be experienced by the patient include:

1   ☐   diarrhoea
2   ☐   headache
3   ☐   dry mouth

A   ☐   1, 2, 3
B   ☐   1, 2 only
C   ☐   2, 3 only
D   ☐   1 only
E   ☐   3 only

Q98   Which is the preferred proprietary product that could be dispensed for clarithromycin?

A   ☐   Klaricid
B   ☐   Miocamen
C   ☐   Zithromax
D   ☐   Erythroped
E   ☐   Rulid

Q99   Losec MUPS:

1   ☐   contains omeprazole
2   ☐   could be dispersed in water or fruit juice
3   ☐   could be chewed

A   ☐   1, 2, 3
B   ☐   1, 2 only
C   ☐   2, 3 only
D   ☐   1 only
E   ☐   3 only

Q100 Prior to prescribing this treatment, which conditions should be excluded?

1   ☐ breast-feeding
2   ☐ gastric carcinoma
3   ☐ *Helicobacter pylori* infection

A   ☐ 1, 2, 3
B   ☐ 1, 2 only
C   ☐ 2, 3 only
D   ☐ 1 only
E   ☐ 3 only

Test 1

Answers

A1 C

Fucicort contains fusidic acid (antibacterial) and betamethasone, which is more potent than hydrocortisone (corticosteroid). Fucidin H contains fusidic acid and hydrocortisone; Daktacort contains miconazole (imidazole antifungal) and hydrocortisone; Canesten HC contains clotrimazole (imidazole antifungal) and hydrocortisone. Hydrocortisyl is a proprietary (trade name) preparation of hydrocortisone.

A2 E

Headache accompanied by loss of consciousness, neck stiffness and neurological signs such as paraesthesia and slurred speech requires referral.

A3 B

Nifedipine is a calcium-channel blocker of the dihydropyridine group. It relaxes smooth muscle and dilates both coronary and peripheral arteries by interfering with the inward displacement of calcium-channel ions through the active cell membrane. Unlike verapamil, nifedipine can be given with beta-blockers. Long-acting formulations of nifedipine are preferred in the long-term treatment of hypertension.

A4 C

In response to the presence of antigenic stimuli, in seasonal allergic rhinitis (hay fever), mast cells and basophils are sensitised and inflammatory mediators, such as leukotrienes and prostaglandins, are released. Osteocytes are bone cells involved in bone formation.

A5   D

Information required in patient medication records includes name, age and gender of the patient, diagnosis, current medication therapies, and medication allergies.

A6   B

Uniflu contains paracetamol, codeine (opioid analagesic), caffeine, diphenydramine (antihistamine), phenylephrine (nasal decongestant) and ascorbic acid. Day Nurse is the closest equivalent to Uniflu, as it contains paracetamol, phenylpropanolamine (nasal decongestant) and dextromethorphan (antitussive). Actifed contains triprolidine (antihistamine) and pseudoephedrine (nasal decongestant). Phenergan and Xyzal contain the antihistamines promethazine and levocetirizine respectively, whereas Ventolin contains salbutamol (adrenoceptor agonist).

A7   A

Odourless vaginal discharge is a common symptom of vaginal candidiasis. Vaginal candidiasis accompanied by abdominal pain and fever warrants referral. Vaginal candidiasis occurring in diabetic patients and during pregnancy indicates referral.

A8   D

Long-term use of stimulant laxatives, such as bisacodyl and senna, precipitates atonic non-functioning colon. In the elderly, constipation generally requires long-term management. Use of magnesium salts as laxatives is indicated when rapid evacuation is required. Long-term use of magnesium salts and liquid paraffin is not recommended. Lactulose is a semi-synthetic disaccharide which can be given on a regular basis to elderly patients as a laxative preparation.

A9   A

Hydralazine is a vasodilator antihypertensive drug. Valsartan and losartan are specific angiotensin-II receptor antagonists, perindopril and enalapril are angiotensin-converting enzyme inhibitors thereby inhibiting the conversion of angiotensin-I into the more potent vasoconstrictor angiotensin-II.

A10   A

Concurrent administration of lithium and selective serotonin re-uptake inhibitors, such as paroxetine, results in an increased risk of central nervous system effects and lithium toxicity.

A11   A

Rofecoxib, a non-steroidal anti-inflammatory drug, is a cyclo-oxygenase-2 selective inhibitor with similar effect to diclofenac. Rofecoxib is not indicated for long-term management of osteoarthritis and does not provide protection against ischaemic cardiovascular events. Rofecoxib which is marketed as Vioxx is contraindicated in patients with active peptic ulceration or gastro-intestinal bleeding. Mobic is the proprietary preparation of meloxicam.

A12   D

Theophylline is a narrow therapeutic drug, plasma concentrations of which must be maintained at 10–20 mg/L. Plasma concentrations above 20 mg/L increase the severity and frequency of adverse effects.

A13   D

Motilium contains domperidone which is a dopamine antagonist and acts on the chemoreceptor trigger zone. It is ineffective in motion sickness. Stugeron contains cinnarizine; Avomine and Phenergan contain promethazine; and Biodramina contains dimenhydrinate. Cinnarizine, promethazine and dimen- hydrinate are all antihistamines indicated in motion sickness.

A14   E

Alfuzosin is a selective alpha-blocker, which relaxes smooth muscle, thereby increasing urinary flow rate. Due to its alpha-blockade, alfuzosin tends to lower the blood pressure and the first dose of the drug may lead to a hypotensive effect.

A15   D

Mupirocin is only available as cream or ointment intended for topical use.

A16   B

Diazepam is a prescription-only medicine whereas pethidine, morphine, alfen- tanil and phenazocine are controlled drugs.

A17   C

Famciclovir, which is the pro-drug of penciclovir, is indicated in acute genital herpes simplex and in the treatment of varicella zoster. Famciclovir is avail- able as tablets. Valaciclovir is the ester of aciclovir.

A18   D

Herpes labialis or cold sores can be precipitated by trauma to the lips and sun- light. In patients whose immune system is compromised, such as in immuno- suppression or in cases of viral infections, herpes labialis may be precipitated. Dental caries do not precipitate cold sores.

A19   B

Soframycin containing the antibacterial framycetin is available both as eye ointment and eye drops. Zovirax containing aciclovir is available as eye ointment only. Fucithalmic containing fusidic acid, Livostin containing levocabastine and Timoptol containing timolol are available as eye drops only.

A20   D

Cilest contains ethinylestradiol and norgestimate whereas Microgynon contains ethinylestradiol in combination with levonorgestrel. Both are combined oral contraceptives available as tablets which have to be taken once daily for 21 days. Both are contraindicated in patients with venous thromboembolic diseases.

A21   C

Hydrocortisyl cream containing hydrocortisone is indicated for the treatment of contact dermatitis. It is applied sparingly once or twice daily for a maximum period of 1 week. Topical antihistamine preparations such as Histergan (diphenhydramine) cream are not recommended as they may cause sensitisation and are only marginally effective. Sedating systemic antihistamines may help but Clarityn tablets would not be the treatment of choice as they contain loratidine which is non-sedating. Preparations containing antifungals such as Pevaryl (econazole) and Travocort (isoconazole, diflucortolone) are of no use in the treatment of contact dermatitis.

A22   D

Buspar containing buspirone is indicated in short-term anxiety. Diazepam, Stilnoct containing zolpidem, Heminevrin containing clomethiazole, and Phenergan containing promethazine are all indicated in insomnia.

A23 C

Rhinocort Aqua and Beconase are preparations containing topical nasal corticosteroids (budesonide and beclometasone (beclomethasone) respectively). Dexa-Rhinaspray Duo is a topical preparation containing a corticosteroid (dexamethasone) and a nasal decongestant (tramazoline). Livostin contains an antihistamine (levocabastine); Otrivine contains a nasal decongestant (xylometazoline); and Rhinocap is a systemic preparation containing a nasal decongestant (phenylephrine), an antihistamine (dimenhydrinate) and caffeine.

A24 B

Bupivacaine is an anaesthetic with a slow onset but a long duration of action. It is indicated for continuous epidural analgesia in labour. Xylocaine is the proprietary preparation of lidocaine (lignocaine). Lidocaine injections are used in dentistry.

A25 D

Haloperidol is indicated for schizophrenia, severe anxiety, motor tics, intractable hiccup and severe anxiety. It is not indicated in the treatment of parkinsonism which may be aggravated through its use, as haloperidol tends to cause extrapyramidal symptoms.

A26 A

Twinrix is a vaccine combining hepatitis A virus units and hepatitis B surface antigen, thereby protecting against hepatitis A and B.

A27 B

ACT-HIB is a *Haemophilus influenzae* type b vaccine. The risk of infection resulting from *H. influenzae* type b decreases after 4 years of age and the vaccine is not required after this age.

A28   D

Fluarix is an influenza vaccine containing the H and N component of the prevalent influenza strains, against which vaccination is recommended each year by the World Health Organization.

A29   B

Constipation is a side-effect of Zofran, which contains ondansetron.

A30   C

Cytotec containing misoprostol (prostaglandin analogue) may cause abnormal vaginal bleeding.

A31   E

Diamox containing acetazolamide (carbonic anhydrase inhibitor) may cause paraesthesia.

A32   E

Aldactone containing spironolactone (potassium-sparing diuretic and an aldosterone antagonist) is used with caution in cases of porphyria.

A33   B

Inderal containing propranolol (beta-adrenoceptor blocking agent) is used with caution in diabetic patients.

A34 B

Inderal containing propranolol (beta-adrenoceptor blocking agent) is used with caution in myasthenia gravis.

A35 D

Nu-Seals containing aspirin is marketed by Lilly.

A36 A

Bricanyl containing terbutaline (selective $beta_2$ agonist bronchodilator) is marketed by AstraZeneca.

A37 C

Alupent containing orciprenaline (non-selective $beta_2$ agonist bronchodilator) is marketed by Boehringer Ingelheim.

A38 C

Difflam containing benzydamine (local analgesic) is available as an oral rinse and is indicated for inflammatory conditions of the oropharynx and for palliative relief in post-radiation mucositis.

A39 B

Livostin containing levocabastine (antihistamine) is available as a nasal spray used in hay fever. It is also available as eye drops.

A40   D

Molcer ear drops containing dioctyl sodium sulphosuccinate is a preparation used to remove ear wax.

A41   C

Liver function tests must be carried out before and within 1–3 months of starting treatment with statins, such as fluvastatin. Liver function tests are thereafter carried out at 6-month intervals for 1 year.

A42   E

Selective serotonin re-uptake inhibitors, such as fluvoxamine, are used with caution in patients with epilepsy and should be discontinued if convulsions occur.

A43   D

Lithium therapy necessitates the monitoring of thyroid function every 6–12 months in stabilised patients. Occurrence of symptoms such as lethargy, which may reflect hypothyroidism, should be monitored.

A44   A

Levodopa must be used with caution in patients with peptic ulcer disease because it may cause gastrointestinal bleeding.

A45   C

Dulcolax containing bisacodyl (stimulant laxative) is available as 5 mg tablets.

A46 B

Zantac containing ranitidine (H_2-receptor antagonist) is available as 75 mg, 150 mg or 300 mg tablets.

A47 D

Phenergan containing promethazine hydrochloride (sedating antihistamine), is available as 10 mg or 25 mg tablets.

A48 A

Imodium containing loperamide (antidiarrhoeal) is available as 2 mg capsules.

A49 D

Mictral is a proprietary preparation of nalidixic acid (quinolone).

A50 A

Noroxin is a proprietary preparation of norfloxacin (quinolone).

A51 B

Relifex is a proprietary preparation of nabumetone (non-steroidal anti-inflammatory drug).

A52 C

Adalat is a proprietary preparation of nifedipine (a dihydropyridine calcium-channel blocker).

A53 E

Acarbose, an antidiabetic that inhibits intestinal alpha glucosidases, may cause flatulence and diarrhoea. The tablets, which can be taken three times daily, must be taken before food.

A54 A

Esomeprazole is a proton pump inhibitor and may cause headache, pruritus and dizziness as side-effects.

A55 B

Digoxin (cardiac glycoside) and trihexyphenidyl (benzhexol) (antimuscarinic drug) must be used with caution in elderly patients. Low doses are recommended in elderly patients to avoid toxicity. Lactulose may be safely administered to elderly patients with constipation.

A56 A

Patients taking mefloquine as prophylaxis against malaria should be advised to take the medication regularly and to avoid mosquito bites. Dizziness may be caused by mefloquine and patients should be informed about this side-effect.

A57 B

Venous thrombosis results in congestion in the affected foot. The foot becomes painful, swollen and blue or black in colour, caused by lack of blood circulation.

A58 B

Blood glucose monitoring measures the concentration at the time of the test. Monitoring in diabetic patients is essential to detect fluctuations in blood glucose concentrations and to help detect hypoglycaemia. Patients should be trained and encouraged to measure their blood glucose concentrations regularly. This would allow for alterations of their insulin dose made once or twice weekly. Insulin dose should not be altered on a daily basis except during illness when patients are under medical supervision.

A59 A

Cancer of the large bowel can present with symptoms of bowel obstruction, such as nausea, vomiting, colicky pain, constipation and abdominal distention. Blood in the stools (melaena) is a classic symptom of colorectal cancer. Cancer of the large bowel may be at an advanced stage before the symptoms are present.

A60 A

Symptoms of tuberculosis, which are mild in the early stages of the disease, include persistent cough, fever and weight loss.

A61 D

Detection of head lice infestation is based on identifying lice by detection combing. Head lice detection cannot be solely based on an itchy scalp because not all children with head lice have the symptom. Furthermore, itchiness is caused by an allergic reaction to the lice, which may develop a few weeks after the infection and can persist for some time after eradication. Infestation is equally likely to occur in clean or dirty hair.

A62 A

Symptoms characteristic of acute bronchitis include chest tightness, cough with purulent sputum, chest soreness, wheeziness, and difficulty in breathing.

A63 A

Tinea pedis or athelete's foot is a fungal infection affecting the feet, classically starting between the fourth and fifth toes but which can spread to other areas of the foot. The classic symptoms include itchiness and redness in the affected area, which later on becomes white, macerated and sore.

A64 C

Interferon beta, which is indicated for multiple sclerosis, is administered parenterally only. The most common side-effects are irritation at the injection site and influenza-like symptoms, such as fever, myalgia, chills and malaise. The side-effects tend to decrease with time.

A65 C

Tamoxifen is an oestrogen-receptor antagonist. It is used in post-menopausal women with oestrogen-receptor-positive metastatic breast cancer at a dose of 20 mg daily. It can also be used in combination with chemotherapy. Severe side-effects are infrequent; however, it is associated with a small risk of endometrial cancer. Patients should be informed and reassured that the benefits of the treatment outweigh the risk.

A66 C

Administration of bromocriptine necessitates monitoring pituitary gland function, especially during pregnancy, whereas in psychotic disorders, including schizophrenia, bromocriptine must be administered with caution. There is no need to reduce the dose or administer bromocriptine with caution in patients with renal impairment.

A67 B

Capecitabine is an antimetabolite neoplastic and cyclophosphamide is an alkylating neoplastic, both of which can be administered orally. Carboplatin is a platinum compound (antineoplastic). All currently available platinum compounds are administered parenterally via the intravenous route.

A68 A

Dydrogesterone is a progesterone analogue. One of its indications is endometriosis, in which case dydrogesterone is administered at a dose of 10 mg two to three times daily. Progestogens are contraindicated in severe liver impairment and in patients with a history of liver tumours.

A69 B

Premarin is a preparation containing conjugated oestrogens indicated to relieve vasomotor symptoms in menopause for women who have undergone hysterectomy. Livial is a preparation containing tibolone. Tibolone combines oestrogenic, progestogenic and weak androgenic activity and helps relieve vasomotor symptoms associated with menopause. Logynon is a combined tricyclic oral contraceptive containing ethinylestradiol and levonorgestrel and is not indicated in menopause.

A70 A

Side-effects associated with testosterone include headache, hirsutism and gynaecomastia.

A71 A

Both levofloxacin and ciprofloxacin are quinolones active against both Gram-negative and Gram-positive bacteria. However, levofloxacin has greater activity against pneumoccocci than ciprofloxacin. Levofloxacin may cause tremor and tachycardia as side-effects. All quinolones should be administered with caution in patients with a history of epilepsy.

A72   C

The description given is typical of verrucas. Verrucas are plantar warts caused by the human papilloma virus affecting the sole of the foot in pressure areas. The lesion is pushed into the epidermis eventually forming a dry hard plaque with a small central black core, which comprises blood vessels. Preparations containing salicylic acid, which is a keratolytic agent, may be used as treatment. Diabetic patients should be referred.

A73   A

Lichen planus is a condition of unknown aetiology presenting as small pruritic and shiny papules, which initially may appear purple in colour. It affects the limbs, wrists, trunk, genitalia and the mouth, in which case ulcerated lesions occur on the gingival tissue. Treatment for lichen planus involves the use of systemic antihistamines but sometimes corticosteroids are required.

A74   C

Chickenpox is caused by the virus herpes zoster which could be contracted from patients with shingles but not vice versa. Calamine lotion or oral sedative antihistamines, such as promethazine, are used to provide relief from the itchy vesicles typical of chickenpox.

A75   B

Terbinafine is the drug of choice in fungal nail infections. Treatment with terbinafine can take up to 6 weeks depending on the condition, with a minimum duration of 2 weeks. Photosensitivity may occur as a side-effect to terbinafine.

A76   B

Anti-lice alcoholic preparations are considered more effective than aqueous preparations. However, alcoholic preparations are unsuitable for use in children and patients with asthma and eczema. Anti-lice preparations should not be used for prophylaxis because they are ineffective and may encourage the development of resistance.

A77   E

Rosiglitazone is a thiazolidinedione that can be used in combination with metformin or a sulphonylurea such as gliclazide. Rosiglitazone should be administered with caution in patients with cardiovascular disease.

A78   A

When compared with soluble insulin, the human analogue insulin aspart has a faster onset and a shorter duration of action, resulting in a higher fasting and preprandial blood glucose concentration. The incidence of hypoglycaemia tends to be lower with insulin aspart than with soluble insulin.

A79   B

Fluconazole is a triazole antifungal that may be administered in recurrent vaginal candidiasis. Fluconazole interacts with sulphonylureas such as glibenclamide, resulting in increased plasma concentrations of the sulphonylurea.

A80   B

Cradle cap is a form of seborrhoeic dermatitis of the scalp affecting babies aged 1–3 months. The condition is not contagious and can be treated by rubbing baby oil into the scalp, leaving it overnight and shampooing afterwards.

A81   B

Oruvail is a proprietary preparation of ketoprofen and Feldene is a proprietary preparation of piroxicam, both of which are non-steroidal anti-inflammatory drugs; Nootropil is a proprietary preparation of piracetam, which is not. Nootropil is indicated as adjunctive treatment in cortical myoclonus.

A82   E

Antibacterial treatment is generally not required in cases of gastroenteritis. Typhoid fever is treated with ciprofloxacin (quinolone), cefotaxime (third generation cephalosporin) or chloramphenicol. Impetigo necessitates the systemic use of flucloxacillin or erythromycin. Topical fusidic acid or mupirocin may also be used.

A83   D

Nappy rash is effectively managed by the application of a barrier preparation, such as zinc and castor oil ointment. Antipruritic creams, such as Anthisan cream, containing the antihistamine mepyramine and Eurax cream, containing crotamiton, are of no use.

A84   D

Paclitaxel is a taxane antineoplastic used in the treatment of primary ovarian cancer.

A85   B

Co-trimoxazole refers to the combination of sulfamethoxazole and trimethoprim, which offers synergistic activity. Co-trimoxazole is associated with rare but serious side-effects, such as Stevens-Johnson syndrome, bone marrow suppression and blood dyscrasias.

A86   B

Pethidine is a less potent opioid analgesic than morphine. Pethidine is not suitable for continuous pain because of its short-lasting analgesia.

A87   D

Minocycline differs from the other tetracyclines in that it is active against *Neisseria meningitidis*. Topical and systemic preparations of tetracyclines are indicated in acne.

A88   C

Zafirlukast is a leukotriene-receptor antagonist. Leukotriene-receptor antagonists are used for prophylaxis of asthma and should not be used to relieve an attack of acute severe asthma.

A89   C

Xenical is a proprietary preparation of orlistat which is used as an adjunct to diet in the treatment of obesity.

A90   A

The active ingredient of Xenical, orlistat, is a pancreatic lipase inhibitor. Side-effects include faecal urgency, liquid oily stools and flatulence. Xenical capsules are administered before, during or up to 1 hour after the two main meals, twice daily.

A91   D

Daktacort cream is a trade name for a preparation containing miconazole (imidazole antifungal) and hydrocortisone (corticosteroid).

A92   D

As Daktacort cream contains hydrocortisone, a mild steroid, its use is rarely associated with side-effects unlike the potent and very potent steroids. The product is generally applied once or twice daily for 1 week. It should be discarded once the expiry date has elapsed. Daktacort is only available as cream or ointment.

A93   A

Daktacort preparations are indicated when patients have fungal infections accompanied by inflammation of the skin.

A94   D

In this case Daktacort cream should be applied sparingly, twice daily for 1 week.

A95   A

The therapy prescribed is a 1-week triple therapy regimen consisting of amoxicillin, clarithromycin and omeprazole against *Helicobacter pylori* infection.

A96   D

Irfen is a proprietary preparation of ibuprofen, a non-steroidal anti-inflammatory drug which, as a side-effect, may cause peptic ulceration. Irfen is contraindicated in patients with active ulceration and the patient is being treated for peptic ulceration. Therefore Irfen should not be used. Clarityn, which contains the non-sedating antihistamine loratidine; and Rennie, which is an antacid containing calcium carbonate and magnesium carbonate, do not cause gastrointestinal bleeding and may be taken by the patient.

A97   A

Headache, diarrhoea and dry mouth are side-effects that may be caused by omeprazole.

A98   A

Klaricid is a proprietary preparation of clarithromycin. Miocamen is a proprietary preparation of midecamycin; Zithromax contains azithromycin; Erythroped contains erythromycin; and Rulid contains roxithromycin.

A99   B

Losec MUPS is a proprietary preparation of omeprazole available as dispersible tablets that can be dispersed either in water or fruit juice. Tablets should not be chewed.

A100 B

Proton pump inhibitors such as omeprazole may mask the symptoms of gastric cancer. Omeprazole is best avoided during breast-feeding. The prescription is indicative of triple therapy used as eradication therapy in *H. pylori* infection.

Test 2

Questions

Questions 1–25

Directions: Each of the questions or incomplete statements is followed by five suggested answers. Select the best answer in each case.

Q1   All of the following products contain aspirin EXCEPT:

- A ☐ Distalgesic
- B ☐ Alka-Seltzer
- C ☐ Anadin Extra
- D ☐ Codis
- E ☐ Aspro

Q2   The management of unstable angina includes all EXCEPT:

- A ☐ aspirin
- B ☐ exercise stress test
- C ☐ anticoagulation
- D ☐ isosorbide dinitrate
- E ☐ nifedipine

Q3   Digoxin:

- A ☐ clearance is by the liver
- B ☐ increases conduction of the AV node
- C ☐ decreases the force of myocardial contraction
- D ☐ has a short half-life
- E ☐ may cause atrial tachycardia in overdosage

Q4 Which of the following causes bronchodilatation?

A ☐ adrenaline (epinephrine)
B ☐ histamine
C ☐ prostaglandin E2
D ☐ kinins
E ☐ guaifenesin

Q5 Information sources recommended to be available in a dispensary include all EXCEPT:

A ☐ *British National Formulary*
B ☐ *Gray's Anatomy*
C ☐ *Martindale: The Complete Drug Reference*
D ☐ pharmacy legislation
E ☐ *Pharmacological Basis of Therapeutics*

Q6 What is an appropriate therapeutic alternative for Clarinase?

A ☐ Cirrus
B ☐ Rhinopront
C ☐ Polaramine
D ☐ Clarityn
E ☐ Telfast

Q7 A patient who is infested with *Enterobius vermicularis* probably has:

A ☐ duodenal haemorrhaging
B ☐ increased urinary output
C ☐ nocturnal perianal pruritus
D ☐ diarrhoea
E ☐ abdominal pain

Q8 A patient asks for an over-the-counter cold remedy. The pharmacist could appropriately suggest:

A ☐ Otrivine drops
B ☐ Beecham's Hot Lemon and Honey powders
C ☐ Rhinopront capsules
D ☐ Actifed Compound Linctus
E ☐ Codipront cum Expectorans syrup

Q9 Which of the following drugs acts by enzyme inhibition?

A ☐ salbutamol
B ☐ acetazolamide
C ☐ tolbutamide
D ☐ chlorpromazine
E ☐ zafirlukast

Q10 A significant clinical interaction may occur if sildenafil is administered concomitantly with:

A ☐ Zantac tablets
B ☐ Tagamet tablets
C ☐ Isordil tablets
D ☐ Augmentin tablets
E ☐ Tenormin tablets

Q11 Famciclovir can be used in the treatment of:

A ☐ chickenpox
B ☐ influenza
C ☐ warts
D ☐ rubella
E ☐ mumps

Q12 The maximum dosage of ergotamine is:

A ☐ 8 mg per day and 12 mg per week

B ☐ 6 mg per day and 20 mg per week

C ☐ 6 mg per day and 15 mg per week

D ☐ 10 mg per day and 10 mg per week

E ☐ 10 mg per day and 6 mg per week

Q13 Appropriate preparations that could be dispensed over-the-counter to treat pruritus associated with an insect bite include all of the following EXCEPT:

A ☐ Systral cream

B ☐ Anthisan cream

C ☐ Histergan cream

D ☐ Hydrocortisyl cream

E ☐ Dermovate cream

Q14 Ergotamine is used as an antimigraine drug because it:

A ☐ is a beta-adrenergic agonist

B ☐ causes vasoconstriction

C ☐ inhibits platelet aggregation

D ☐ causes elevation of the pain threshold

E ☐ is a prostaglandin antagonist

Q15 For the intravenous administration of hydrocortisone, a suitable formulation is:

A ☐ base

B ☐ acetate

C ☐ propionate

D ☐ cypionate

E ☐ sodium succinate

Q16 A product that should be refrigerated during storage in the pharmacy is:

A ☐ Spersallerg eye drops
B ☐ Otosporin ear drops
C ☐ Garamycin eye drops
D ☐ Hydrocortisyl cream
E ☐ Cerumol ear drops

Q17 The site of action of Lasix is at the:

A ☐ distal tubule
B ☐ proximal tubule
C ☐ collecting duct
D ☐ loop of Henle
E ☐ glomerular membrane

Q18 All of the following skin disorders are worsened by sun exposure EXCEPT:

A ☐ seborrhoeic dermatitis
B ☐ furuncles
C ☐ chloasma
D ☐ acne vulgaris
E ☐ herpes simplex labialis

Q19 Drugs that are commercially available in more than one strength include all EXCEPT:

A ☐ Distaclor capsules
B ☐ Istin tablets
C ☐ Inderal tablets
D ☐ Naprosyn capsules
E ☐ Migril tablets

Q20 Triamcinolone differs from hydrocortisone in that it:

A ☐ is less potent as an anti-inflammatory

B ☐ is available in the oral dosage form

C ☐ has a longer duration of action

D ☐ has more mineralocorticoid activity

E ☐ is available for topical application

Q21 What is the most appropriate treatment for a mycotic vaginal super-infection?

A ☐ Betadine douche

B ☐ Ortho-Gynest cream

C ☐ Fulcin tablets

D ☐ Gyno-Daktarin pessary

E ☐ Canesten cream

Q22 Which of the following products is NOT indicated as an agent to be used in gastrointestinal ulcer healing?

A ☐ omeprazole

B ☐ rabeprazole

C ☐ misoprostol

D ☐ loperamide

E ☐ ranitidine

Q23 Which of the following products may be recommended as an equivalent to Proctosedyl oinment?

A ☐ Preparation H

B ☐ Xyloproct

C ☐ Anacal

D ☐ Nupercainal

E ☐ Anusol

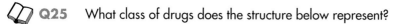

Q24 Cradle cap:

A ☐ is a form of seborrhoeic dermatitis
B ☐ occurs in children over 1 year
C ☐ may be treated initially with corticosteroid scalp application
D ☐ is a lifelong condition
E ☐ is a form of food allergy

Q25 What class of drugs does the structure below represent?

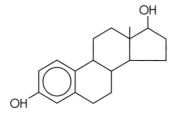

A ☐ oestrogens
B ☐ phenothiazines
C ☐ non-steroidal anti-inflammatory drugs
D ☐ antidepressants
E ☐ glucocorticoids

Questions 26–52

Directions: Each group of questions below consists of five lettered headings followed by a list of numbered questions. For each numbered question select the one heading that is most closely related to it. Each heading may be used once, more than once, or not at all.

Questions 26–28 concern the following manufacturers:

A   ❑ Bayer
B   ❑ Novartis
C   ❑ GlaxoSmithKline
D   ❑ AstraZeneca
E   ❑ Janssen-Cilag

Select, from **A** to **E**, which one of the above manufacturers is associated with the trademarked product:

Q26   Daktarin cream

Q27   Otrivine drops

Q28   Rhinocort Aqua

Questions 29–31 concern the following products:

A   ❑ Buscopan
B   ❑ Zaditen
C   ❑ Aspro
D   ❑ Natrilix
E   ❑ Lescol

Select, from **A** to **E**, the product that should be used with caution in each of the following conditions:

Q29   prostatic hypertrophy

Q30   asthma

Q31   gout

Questions 32–34 concern the following life-threatening adverse reactions:

A ☐ agranulocytosis

B ☐ pseudomembranous colitis

C ☐ respiratory depression

D ☐ cardiovascular collapse

E ☐ nephrotoxicity

Select, from **A** to **E**, the adverse reaction that may occur following administration of the following drugs:

Q32 acetazolamide

Q33 ampicillin

Q34 atracurium

Questions 35–37 concern the following drugs:

A ☐ doxorubicin

B ☐ methotrexate

C ☐ mitomycin

D ☐ cyclophosphamide

E ☐ tamoxifen

Select, from **A** to **E**, which one of the above:

Q35 is limited in its clinical usefulness by cardiotoxicity

Q36 may be used in severe resistant psoriasis

Q37 has a mechanism of action involving alkylation

Questions 38–40 concern the following products:

A ☐ Distalgesic
B ☐ Anadin Extra
C ☐ Cerumol
D ☐ Rinstead
E ☐ Optrex

Select, from A to E, which one of the above:

Q38 has astringent properties

Q39 is co-proxamol

Q40 contains caffeine

Questions 41–44 concern the following drugs:

A ☐ sumatriptan
B ☐ ondansetron
C ☐ tramadol
D ☐ cyclizine
E ☐ pizotifen

Select, from A to E, which one of the above:

Q41 is used in the treatment of acute migraine

Q42 is an opioid analgesic

Q43 should not be used in ischaemic heart disease

Q44 is a specific serotonin antagonist

Questions 45–48 concern the following strengths:

A ☐ 5%
B ☐ 2%
C ☐ 20%
D ☐ 0.05%
E ☐ 10%

Select, from **A** to **E**, a strength in which the following products are available:

Q45 aciclovir cream

Q46 mupirocin ointment

Q47 azelaic acid

Q48 fluticasone cream

Questions 49–52 concern the following drugs:

A ☐ mebeverine
B ☐ mebendazole
C ☐ meloxicam
D ☐ meprobamate
E ☐ maprotiline

Select, from **A** to **E**, which one of the above corresponds to the drug brand name:

Q49 Mobic

Q50 Vermox

Q51 Colofac

Q52 Ludiomil

Questions 53–83

Directions: For each of the questions below, ONE or MORE of the responses is (are) correct. Decide which of the responses is (are) correct. Then choose:

A   ❏ if 1, 2 and 3 are correct
B   ❏ if 1 and 2 only are correct
C   ❏ if 2 and 3 only are correct
D   ❏ if 1 only is correct
E   ❏ if 3 only is correct

Directions summarised				
A	B	C	D	E
1, 2, 3	1, 2 only	2, 3 only	1 only	3 only

Q53   When dispensing alfuzosin hydrochloride, the patient should be advised to:

1   ❏ take the first dose at night before retiring to bed
2   ❏ be careful when driving
3   ❏ avoid alcoholic drink

Q54   Side-effects of venlafaxine include:

1   ❏ diarrhoea
2   ❏ blurred vision
3   ❏ headache

Q55   Care should be taken with the use of the following drugs in a patient with renal impairment:

1   ☐ aciclovir
2   ☐ amoxicillin
3   ☐ naproxen

Q56   When dispensing phenytoin, the patient should be advised:

1   ☐ to keep taking the medicine routinely as directed
2   ☐ to report promptly symptoms of bruising or unexplained bleeding
3   ☐ that visual symptoms commonly occur

Q57   Symptoms of endometriosis include:

1   ☐ infertility
2   ☐ vaginal discharge
3   ☐ pelvic pain a few days after termination of menstruation

Q58   Which of the following vaccines are usually started before 6 months of age?

1   ☐ polio vaccine
2   ☐ pertussis vaccine
3   ☐ BCG vaccine

Q59   Gastro-oesophageal reflux in infants:

1   ☐ usually requires surgical intervention
2   ☐ is extremely rare
3   ☐ may be alleviated by thickening feeds

Q60 Clinical signs of dehydration in children include:

1. ☐ tachycardia
2. ☐ loss of skin turgor
3. ☐ dry tongue

Q61 Clinical features of mumps include:

1. ☐ enlargement of parotid glands
2. ☐ fever
3. ☐ bronchitis

Q62 Which symptoms are characteristic of allergic rhinitis?

1. ☐ shortness of breath
2. ☐ conjunctival lacrimation
3. ☐ prolonged sneezing attacks

Q63 Symptoms of cataracts include:

1. ☐ ocular pain
2. ☐ watery eyes
3. ☐ reduction in visual acuity

Q64 Calcipotriol:

1. ☐ may cause skin discoloration
2. ☐ is a vitamin D derivative
3. ☐ is used for psoriasis

Q65 Ciclosporin:

1. ☐ may cause nephrotoxicity
2. ☐ is associated with gastrointestinal disturbances
3. ☐ is only available as a parenteral preparation

Q66 Ciprofloxacin should be used with caution in:

1 ☐ epileptic patients
2 ☐ children
3 ☐ pregnancy

Q67 Which of the following drugs should be swallowed whole, not chewed?

1 ☐ Arthrotec tablets
2 ☐ Voltarol Retard tablets
3 ☐ Dulcolax tablets

Q68 Ranitidine:

1 ☐ interferes significantly with concomitant warfarin therapy
2 ☐ has maximum maintenance dose for reflux oesophagitis of 150 mg at night
3 ☐ reduces gastric acid output

Q69 Which of the following drugs could cause nausea and vomiting as a side-effect?

1 ☐ prednisolone
2 ☐ omeprazole
3 ☐ paclitaxel

Q70 Side-effects associated with levodopa include:

1 ☐ insomnia
2 ☐ discoloration of urine
3 ☐ headache

Q71 Levocabastine:

1 ☐ may be used for allergic conjunctivitis
2 ☐ is available as a nasal spray
3 ☐ should be applied six times daily

Q72 A patient presents at the pharmacy with a headache that is constantly painful and seems to be worse in the morning:

1. ☐ patient should be asked about a medical history of hypertension
2. ☐ referral should be considered if episode is accompanied by fever, neck stiffness
3. ☐ the headache is characteristically tumorigenic

Q73 Periodontitis:

1. ☐ involves the peritoneum
2. ☐ requires referral
3. ☐ is an inflammatory condition

Q74 In cysitis:

1. ☐ the use of alkalinising agents as a treatment modality is associated with a clinically significant risk of hyperkalaemia
2. ☐ *Escherichia coli* is the most common cause
3. ☐ occurrence in children warrants referral

Q75 Tamoxifen:

1. ☐ is an oestrogen-receptor agonist
2. ☐ common side-effects expected include alopecia, uterine fibroids
3. ☐ is used as adjuvant hormonal treatment in breast cancer

Q76 Nicotine chewing gum in smoking cessation:

1. ☐ provides a residual nicotine level
2. ☐ requires one chewing gum for a minimum of 1 hour
3. ☐ may have aphthous ulceration as a side-effect

Q77   Zolpidem:

1   ☐ is a benzodiazepine
2   ☐ has a long duration of action
3   ☐ should be used with caution in patients with hepatic impairment

Q78   Orciprenaline:

1   ☐ is available only as a metered dose inhaler
2   ☐ is a selective beta$_2$ adrenoceptor stimulant
3   ☐ can be prescribed for a child aged 4 years

Q79   Gliclazide:

1   ☐ when administered concomitantly with fluconazole, results in a lower plasma concentration of gliclazide
2   ☐ is a sulphonylurea
3   ☐ has a shorter half-life than glibenclamide

Q80   Which of the following statements about typhoid fever is (are) true?

1   ☐ it is caused by a coccus
2   ☐ it has an incubation period of 4 weeks
3   ☐ it may be associated with rose spots

Q81   Examples of antipsychotic drugs include:

1   ☐ Largactil
2   ☐ Serenace
3   ☐ Tegretol

Q82   For which of the following infections is prophylaxis undertaken by means of a vaccination program?

1   ☐ hepatitis B
2   ☐ malaria
3   ☐ hepatitis C

Q83 The following are effective in the management of fungal nail infections:

1 ☐ griseofulvin
2 ☐ terbinafine
3 ☐ nystatin

Questions 84–88

Directions: The following questions consist of a first statement followed by a second statement. Decide whether the first statement is true or false. Decide whether the second statement is true or false. Then choose:

A ☐ if both statements are true and the second statement is a *correct explanation* of the first statement

B ☐ if both statements are true but the second statement *is NOT a correct explanation* of the first statement

C ☐ if the first statement is true but the second statement is false

D ☐ if the first statement is false but the second statement is true

E ☐ if both statements are false

Q84 Orlistat is an enzyme inhibitor. Orlistat should be taken three times

Directions summarised			
	First statement	**Second statement**	
A	True	True	Second statement is a *correct explanation* of the first
B	True	True	Second statement is *NOT a correct explanation* of the first
C	True	False	
D	False	True	
E	False	False	

daily.

Q85 Enalapril may precipitate a hypoglycaemic attack in a diabetic patient. Enalapril may potentiate the effect of sulphonylureas.

Q86 Repaglinide stimulates peripheral utilisation of glucose. Repaglinide is indicated only as monotherapy of diabetes mellitus.

Q87 Urinalysis for glucose monitoring is a good indicator of hypoglycaemia or hyperglycaemia. Blood glucose concentrations should be maintained at a constant level.

Q88 100 μg of budesonide are equivalent to 200 μg of fluticasone. Budesonide and fluticasone are both indicated for the prophylaxis of allergic rhinitis.

Questions 89-100

Directions: These questions involve cases. Read the prescription or case and answer the questions.

Questions 89-90: Use the prescription below:

Patient's name   ....

Xalatan drops
1 drop o.n.   m. 1 bottle

Doctor's signature   ....

Q89 For which of these conditions are these eye drops prescribed?

A ☐ cataracts
B ☐ glaucoma
C ☐ blepharitis
D ☐ conjunctivitis
E ☐ iritis

Q90 Xalatan:

1 ☐ is a prostaglandin analogue
2 ☐ may cause eye discoloration
3 ☐ is administered once daily

A ☐ 1, 2, 3
B ☐ 1, 2 only
C ☐ 2, 3 only
D ☐ 1 only
E ☐ 3 only

Question 91–94: Use the prescription below:

Patient's name	....
Benzamycin gel	
b.d. m. 1 bottle	
Doctor's signature	....

Q91 The active ingredient(s) of Benzamycin is (are):

A ⬜ azelaic acid
B ⬜ benzoyl peroxide
C ⬜ benzoyl peroxide, erythromycin
D ⬜ benzoyl peroxide, clindamycin
E ⬜ erythromycin

Q92 Adverse effects associated with Benzamycin include:

1 ⬜ redness
2 ⬜ stinging
3 ⬜ blistering of the skin

A ⬜ 1, 2, 3
B ⬜ 1, 2 only
C ⬜ 2, 3 only
D ⬜ 1 only
E ⬜ 3 only

Q93 Benzamycin is prescribed when the patient has:

A ⬜ verrucas
B ⬜ corns
C ⬜ acne
D ⬜ fungal infection
E ⬜ bacterial infection

Q94   When dispensing Benzamycin, the pharmacist should:

1   ☐ reconstitute the product
2   ☐ advise the patient to avoid sunlight
3   ☐ advise the patient to apply gel freely

A   ☐ 1, 2, 3
B   ☐ 1, 2 only
C   ☐ 2, 3 only
D   ☐ 1 only
E   ☐ 3 only

Question 95–100: Use the patient profile below:

Patient medication file

Patient's name   ....

Age   63 years

Allergies   none

Diagnosis   hypertension, arthritis, anxiety

Medication record   bendroflumethiazide (bendrofluazide) 2.5 mg daily
                    Zestril 10 mg daily
                    Valium 5 mg t.d.s.
                    Deltacortril 10 mg daily
                    methotrexate 2.5 mg as directed
                    paracetamol 500 mg prn

Q95 Patients taking bendroflumethiazide (bendrofluazide) are often given a potassium supplement. The patient may not need one because she is also taking:

A ☐ Valium
B ☐ Zestril
C ☐ Deltacortril
D ☐ methotrexate
E ☐ paracetamol

Q96 When dispensing the medications, the pharmacist should advise the patient against the concomitant use of:

1 ☐ Maalox
2 ☐ alcohol
3 ☐ Voltarol

A ☐ 1, 2, 3
B ☐ 1, 2 only
C ☐ 2, 3 only
D ☐ 1 only
E ☐ 3 only

Q97 Patient should contact doctor if cough develops because:

1 ☐ methotrexate may cause pulmonary toxicity
2 ☐ it indicates need of an antibacterial drug
3 ☐ it may indicate adrenal suppression

A ☐ 1, 2, 3
B ☐ 1, 2 only
C ☐ 2, 3 only
D ☐ 1 only
E ☐ 3 only

Q98 Which of the following laboratory tests should be performed while the patient is taking methotrexate?

1 ☐ liver function tests
2 ☐ full blood count
3 ☐ renal function tests

A ☐ 1, 2, 3
B ☐ 1, 2 only
C ☐ 2, 3 only
D ☐ 1 only
E ☐ 3 only

Q99 The patient is instructed to take methotrexate:

A ☐ daily
B ☐ twice daily
C ☐ every alternate day
D ☐ weekly
E ☐ monthly

Q100 Disadvantages of Deltacortril therapy include:

1 ☐ precipitation of osteoporosis
2 ☐ insomnia
3 ☐ candidiasis

A ☐ 1, 2, 3
B ☐ 1, 2 only
C ☐ 2, 3 only
D ☐ 1 only
E ☐ 3 only

Test 2

Answers

A1   A

Distalgesic is a combination analgesic containing the combination known as co-proxamol, made up of paracetamol and dextropropoxyphene, the latter being a mild opioid analgesic. Alka-Seltzer is presented as effervescent tablets containing aspirin, citric acid and sodium bicarbonate. Anadin Extra is a combination analgesic containing aspirin, paracetamol and caffeine (a weak stimulant). Codis is also an analgesic preparation combining aspirin and codeine. Aspro is an effervescent preparation of aspirin.

A2   B

Unstable angina is distinguished from stable angina by changes in frequency and severity of attacks. The aims of the management of angina are to provide supportive care and relief during an acute attack, and to prevent subsequent myocardial infarction and death. Patients should be admitted to hospital and drug therapy optimised. The management involves the administration of aspirin for its antiplatelet effect. Anticoagulation therapy, such as heparin, may also be given. Nitrates, for example, isosorbide dinitrate, are used to relieve ischaemic pain and act as vasodilators. Calcium-channel blockers, such as nifedipine, which are vasodilators, may also be used. Patients are advised to avoid strenuous exercise (and therefore avoid undertaking the exercise stress test) to minimise the occurrence of attacks.

A3   E

Digoxin is a positive inotrope, hence it increases the force of myocardial contraction and may be effective in heart failure. It is a cardiac glycoside, which reduces the conductivity of the atrioventricular (AV) node and which may be used in atrial fibrillation. Digoxin has a long half-life and is given once daily. It is cleared by the renal system and hence renal impairment requires the reduction of digoxin dose. Arrhythmias, such as atrial tachycardia, may be a sign of digoxin toxicity. Digoxin toxicity is enhanced if there are electrolyte disturbances, especially hypokalaemia, hypomagnesaemia and hypercalcaemia.

A4   A

Adrenaline (epinephrine) is a sympathomimetic agent that causes bronchodilation. It is used to relieve bronchospasm in anaphylactic shock reactions. Histamine, kinins and prostaglandins, such as prostaglandin E_2, are inflammatory mediators. In response to allergic stimuli, inflammatory mediators may cause bronchoconstrictions. Guaifenesin is an expectorant preparation that increases bronchial secretions to promote the expulsion of the mucus coughed up.

A5   B

Information sources recommended to be available in a pharmacy include a recent copy of a drug formulary, such as the *British National Formulary;* a current edition of a drug compendium, such as *Martindale: The Complete Drug Reference;* a copy of a pharmacology and therapeutics reference, such us Goodman and Gilman's *Pharmacological Basis of Therapeutics* and an updated copy of the laws regulating the pharmacy profession.

A6   A

Clarinase contains the non-sedating antihistamine loratidine and the nasal decongestant pseudoephedrine. Similarly to Clarinase, Cirrus contains a non-sedating antihistamine cetirizine and the nasal decongestant pseudoephedrine. Rhinopront contains the sedating antihistamine carbinoxamine and the nasal decongestant phenylephrine. Clarityn contains only the non-sedating antihistamine loratidine. Telfast contains only the non-sedating antihistamine fexofenadine.

A7   C

Threadworm infections are caused by *Enterobius vermicularis*. The infestation starts when the patient ingests the worm's ova, which then hatch and infect the small intestine. The female threadworms migrate to the caecum and anus so that at night they lay their eggs in the perianal area. The eggs produce a sticky secretion and attach themselves to the skin. It is the sticky secretion that causes the itchiness which is the main symptom. Enterobiasis, as the condition is known, is treated with the administration of anthelmintics. A single dose is administered. However, as re-infestation is common, a second dose given after 2–3 weeks is recommended. A warm bath taken first thing in the morning is often recommended to remove ova laid during the night.

A8   B

Cold remedies aim to relieve cold symptoms and very often contain a combination of an analgesic, a sedating antihistamine, a nasal decongestant and ascorbic acid. Beecham's Hot Lemon and Honey sachets are a cold remedy preparation containing paracetamol, ascorbic acid and the nasal decongestant phenylephrine. Otrivine drops are a topical preparation containing the nasal decongestant xylometazoline. It is indicated for nasal congestion. Rhinopront capsules contain the sedating antihistamine, carbinoxamine and the nasal decongestant, phenylephrine. Actifed Compound Linctus is a cough preparation containing the sedating antihistamine triprolidine, the nasal decongestant pseudoephedrine and the cough suppressant dextromethorphan. It is therefore indicated in dry cough. Codipront cum Expectorans syrup contains the sedating antihistamine phenyltoloxamine, the cough suppressant codeine phosphate and the expectorant guaifenesin.

A9   B

Acetazolamide is a carbonic anhydrase inhibitor that reduces aqueous humour production and is therefore indicated in glaucoma to reduce the intra-ocular pressure. Salbutamol is a selective, short-acting beta$_2$ agonist used as a bronchodilator in asthma. Tolbutamide is a short-acting sulphonylurea used in type 2 (non-insulin dependent) diabetes mellitus. Chlorpromazine is an aliphatic neuroleptic antipsychotic drug used in schizophrenia. Zafirlukast is a leukotriene-receptor antagonist which is indicated in the prophylaxis of asthma but should not be used to relieve acute severe asthma.

A10   C

Isordil is a proprietary (trade name) preparation of isosorbide dinitrate, a nitrate. Sildenafil, the active ingredient of Viagra, interacts with nitrates and the two active ingredients should not be administered concurrently, as a significant hypotensive effect may occur.

A11   A

Famciclovir is the prodrug of penciclovir and is indicated in the treatment of chickenpox and genital herpes.

A12   A

Ergotamine (ergot alkaloid) is indicated in the treatment of acute migraine. The maximum dose is 8 mg a day and 12 mg a week.

A13   E

Topical antihistamines and topical corticosteroid preparations are indicated to treat pruritus associated with insect bites. Systral cream contains the topical anithistamine chlorphenoxamine; Anthisan cream contains the antihistamine mepyramine; Histergan cream contains the antihistamine diphenhydramine. Hydrocortisyl cream contains the corticosteroid hydrocortisone. Dermovate is a prescription-only medication containing clobetasol, a very potent steroid used in severe inflammatory skin disorders.

A14 B

Ergotamine is an ergot alkaloid indicated in the treatment of migraine. Ergotamine has marked vasoconstrictor effects.

A15 E

Hydrocortisone for intravenous administration is available as the sodium succinate salt.

A16 B

Otosporin ear drops containing the antibacterials neomycin (aminoglycoside), polymyxin B (polymyxin antibiotic) and the corticosteroid hydrocortisone should be refrigerated. Spersallerg eye drops containing antazoline (anithist-amine) and tetryzoline (decongestant); Garamycin eye drops containing the antibacterial gentamicin (aminoglycoside); Hydrocortisyl cream containing the corticosteroid hydrocortisone; and Cerumol ear drops containing arachis oil, paradichlorobenzene and chlorobutanol, can all be stored at room temperature.

A17 D

Lasix containing furosemide (frusemide) is classified as a loop diuretic and acts by inhibiting re-absorption from the ascending part of the loop of Henle. Thiazide diuretics, such as bendroflumethiazide (bendrofluazide), act by inhibiting re-absorption at the beginning of the distal convoluted tubule.

A18 B

Unlike seborrhoeic dermatitis, chloasma, acne vulgaris and herpes simplex labialis, furuncles (boils) are not worsened by skin exposure.

A19   E

Distaclor (cefaclor, first generation cephalosporin) is available as Distaclor 125 mg/5 mL suspension, 250 mg/5 mL suspension, 250 mg capsules and 500 mg capsules. Istin (amlodipine, a dihydropyridine calcium-channel blocker) is available as Istin 5 mg and 10 mg tablets. Inderal (propranolol, a non-selective fat-soluble beta-blocker) is available as Inderal 10 mg, 40 mg and 80 mg tablets. Naprosyn (naproxen, a non-steroidal anti-inflammatory drug) is available as Naprosyn 250 mg and 500 mg capsules. Migril, the antimigraine tablets contain ergotamine 2 mg (ergot alkaloid), cyclizine 50 mg (antihistamine with anti-emetic properties) and caffeine 100 mg (weak stimulant).

A20   C

Triamcinolone is a corticosteroid that is more potent than hydrocortisone and has a longer duration of action. Triamcinolone has only slight mineralocorticoid activity, whereas hydrocortisone has high mineralocorticoid activity and therefore triamcinolone is unsuitable for disease suppression on a long-term basis. Triamcinolone is available as injection, dental paste, nasal spray and as cream or ointment preparations. Hydrocortisone is available as cream, tablets and injections.

A21   D

Vaginal infections caused by fungi (vaginal candidiasis) are best treated with topical preparations containing imidazoles. Generally, pessaries are preferred to cream formulations. Gyno-Daktarin pessary contains miconazole (imidazole antifungal). Canesten cream containing clotrimazole (imidazole antifungal) would be an alternative to the pessary. In case of recurrence, a single dose of oral fluconazole (triazole antifungal) 150 mg capsule (Diflucan) may be effective. Betadine douche containing povidone-iodine is less effective than the imidazole preparations. Ortho-Gynest cream contains estriol, which is used in vaginal atrophy in post-menopausal women. Fulcin tablets containing griseofulvin are not effective in vaginal candidiasis.

A22   D

Omeprazole and rabeprazole inhibit gastric acid formation by blocking the hydrogen–potassium ATPase pump hence the name proton pump inhibitors. Misoprostol is a synthetic prostaglandin analogue having antisecretory properties, thus helping in the healing of gastric ulcers. Misoprostol is used in elderly patients taking non-steroidal anti-inflammatory drugs and in patients in whom the non-steroidal anti-inflammatory drugs cannot be discontinued. Ranitidine decreases the gastric acid output by antagonising the histamine H_2-receptor. Proton pump inhibitors, misoprostol and H_2-receptor antagonists can all be used in the treatment and prophylaxis of gastric ulcers. Loperamide is an antidiarrhoeal agent.

A23   B

All the preparations are used to soothe haemorrhoids. Procotsedyl ointment contains cinchocaine (anaesthetic) and hydrocortisone (corticosteroid). Xyloproct contains lidocaine (lignocaine; anaesthetic), hydrocortisone (corticosteroid) and aluminium acetate and zinc oxide as astringents. Anacal contains heparinoid and laureth '9'. Nupercainal contains cinchocaine only. Preparation H contains shark liver oil and yeast cell extract only. Anusol contains bismuth, Peru balsam and zinc oxide as astringents. The preparation that, like Proctosedyl, contains an anaesthetic and a corticosteroid, is Xyloproct.

A24   A

Cradle cap is a form of seborrhoeic dermatitis of the scalp presenting in babies up to 3 months of age. The condition appears as scales and crusts on the baby's scalp. It is not contagious and although it may tend to affect babies with a predisposition to food allergy, cradle cap is not a food allergy. The condition, which may be associated with nappy rash, resolves spontaneously within a year. First-line treatment is the application of almond oil, arachis oil or baby oil onto the scalp, leaving it overnight and then washing off the next day.

A25   A

The structure is an 18-carbon steroid and represents estradiol, an oestrogen.

A26   E

Daktarin cream containing the imidazole antifungal miconazole, is a brand marketed by Janssen-Cilag.

A27   B

Otrivine drops containing the nasal decongestant xylometazoline, is a brand marketed by Novartis.

A28   D

Rhinocort Aqua is the proprietary preparation of a topical nasal spray containing the corticosteroid budesonide and is marketed by AstraZeneca.

A29   A

Buscopan contains hyoscine butylbromide, which is a quaternary ammonium compound with antimuscarinic properties. It is used as an antispasmodic and therefore may be useful in irritable bowel syndrome. Hyoscine butylbromide, as with all antimuscarinics, must be used with caution in patients with prostatic hypertrophy, as they may lead to urinary retention, which is avoided in prostatic hypertrophy.

A30   C

Aspro is a proprietary preparation of aspirin (or acetylsalicylic acid). Aspirin, like all the non-steroidal anti-inflammatory drugs, may lead to broncho-constriction and therefore must be used with caution in asthma.

A31   D

Natrilix is a proprietary preparation of indapamide, a thiazide diuretic and hence may cause gout as a side-effect.

A32   A

Acetazolamide is a carbonic anhydrase inhibitor, used primarily in glaucoma to reduce aqueous humour production. Acetazolamide may cause blood disorders including agranulocytosis (deficiency of neutrophils) as a side-effect.

A33   B

Ampicillin is a broad spectrum penicillin antibiotic. Antibiotics tend to cause pseudomembranous colitis as a result of colonisation of the colon by *Clostridium difficile* following antibiotic therapy.

A34   C

Atracurium is a non-depolarising muscle relaxant, which may cause respiratory depression as a side-effect.

A35   A

Doxorubicin is a chemotherapeutic anthracycline antibiotic, which may cause cardiotoxicity through the free-radical mechanism. Cardiotoxicity limits the clinical usefulness as a result of which doxorubicin has a total cumulative dose of about 450 mg/m^2 body surface area. Patients with pre-existing cardiac disease, elderly patients and patients who have received myocardial irradiation must be treated cautiously and cardiac monitoring may be required.

A36 B

Methotrexate is an antimetabolite chemotherapeutic agent, which may also be used for severe resistant psoriasis. The dose is usually 10–25 mg methotrexate administered orally once a week. Haematological and biochemical parameters are monitored throughout treatment.

A37 D

Cyclophosphamide is an antineoplastic agent which causes DNA cross-linking and abnormal base-pairing through a mechanism called alkylation, hence the name alkylating agent. Cyclophosphamide may also be used in resistant rheumatoid arthritis.

A38 E

Optrex preparations contain witch hazel, which has both astringent and anti-inflammatory properties. It is indicated for sore and tired eyes.

A39 A

Distalgesic is a proprietary preparation of co-proxamol, a combination of paracetamol and the mild opioid analgesic dextropropoxyphene.

A40 B

Anadin Extra contains paracetamol, aspirin and caffeine, the latter being a mild stimulant that increases the absorption and activity of the analgesics, paracetamol and aspirin.

A41   A

Sumatriptan is a $5HT_1$ agonist, which is indicated in the treatment of acute migraine attacks. Sumatriptan may cause vasoconstriction as a side-effect and therefore its use is reserved for patients in whom other conventional migraine analgesics have failed.

A42   C

Tramadol is an opioid analgesic, which acts by exerting an opioid effect and through the stimulation of adrenergic and serotonin pathways. Compared with the other opioids, tramadol is less likely to cause the typical opioid side-effects, such as respiratory depression, and constipation. It is also less likely to cause addiction.

A43   A

Sumatriptan, a $5HT_1$ agonist, is contraindicated in ischaemic heart disease as it may cause vasoconstriction, leading to chest tightness, and precipitating ischaemic heart disease.

A44   B

Ondansetron is a $5HT_3$ antagonist, blocking serotonin receptors in the central nervous system and the gastrointestinal tract. It is useful in the management of postoperative nausea and vomiting associated with cytotoxics.

A45   A

The antiviral aciclovir cream is available as 5%. It is indicated in the treatment of herpes simplex infections.

A46   B

Mupirocin is a broad spectrum antibiotic available as a 2% ointment.

A47   C

Azelaic acid, which has antimicrobial and anticomedonal properties, is available as 20% cream indicated for use in acne.

A48   D

Fluticasone cream is a corticosteroid preparation available as 0.05%.

A49   C

Mobic is the proprietary preparation of meloxicam, a non-steroidal anti-inflammatory drug, which is also a selective inhibitor of cyclo-oxygenase-2. It is therefore less likely to cause gastrointestinal side-effects than other non-steroidal anti-inflammatory drugs. However it is still best to administer meloxicam after food.

A50   B

Vermox is the proprietary preparation of mebendazole, which is an anthelmintic. A single dose of mebendazole is indicated in the management of threadworms, with a second dose 2–3 weeks later avoiding re-infection, which tends to be common.

A51   A

Colofac is the proprietary preparation of mebeverine which is an antispasmodic useful in irritable bowel syndrome. Mebeverine is a direct relaxant of the smooth muscle and unlike hyoscine it is not an antimuscarinic.

A52   E

Ludiomil is the proprietary preparation of maprotiline, a heterocyclic antidepressant particularly useful where sedation is required.

A53   B

Alfuzosin is a selective alpha$_1$ blocker, which relaxes the smooth muscle in benign prostatic hyperplasia and hence increases the urinary outflow. Alpha-blockers tend to cause vasodilation leading to hypotension especially after the first dose. Subsequently patients on alpha-blockers are advised to take the first dose at night before retiring to bed. Alpha-blockers also tend to cause drowsiness so patients are advised to be careful when driving.

A54   E

Venlafaxine is a serotonin and noradrenaline (norepinephrine) re-uptake inhibitor indicated in depression and may be used in generalised anxiety disorder. Venlafaxine lacks antimuscarinic side-effects associated with tricyclic antidepressants and hence does not cause blurred vision. It does not cause diarrhoea but may cause headache.

A55   A

The dose of aciclovir in patients with renal impairment should be reduced as aciclovir is eliminated by the renal system. Most penicillins are eliminated by the renal system and hence dose reduction of amoxicillin is required in cases of renal impairment. Non-steroidal anti-inflammatory drugs cause the inhibition of the biosynthesis of prostaglandins involved in the maintenance of renal blood flow. This may precipitate acute renal insufficiency in patients with renal impairment. Furthermore non-steroidal anti-inflammatory drugs tend to cause water and sodium retention and hence aggrevate renal impairment.

A56 B

Phenytoin is an anti-epileptic drug. Patients taking anti-epileptic drugs are advised to take the medicine routinely, as directed, to stabilise and to avoid epileptic attacks as much as possible. Phenytoin has a narrow therapeutic index so it is important to identify side-effects. It may cause blood disorders. Patients are therefore advised to report immediately any symptoms of bruising or unexplained bleeding. Visual symptoms as a result of phenytoin do not commonly occur. Their occurrence may indicate overdosage.

A57 D

Endometriosis refers to the abnormal presence of endometrial tissue growing outside the uterus in places such as the abdomen, the peritoneum, ovary and the bladder. Symptoms of endometriosis include infertility. Pelvic pain may occur before or during menses.

A58 B

The polio vaccine is administered in three doses at 1-month intervals, starting from the age of 2 months. The pertussis vaccine is given in combination with the diphtheria and tetanus vaccines as a 3-in-1 vaccine, the DTP vaccine. The DTP vaccine follows the schedule of the polio vaccine, so at 2 months, the DTP and the polio vaccine are given. Both are repeated at 3 months of age and at 4 months of age. The BCG vaccine is not usually recommended for infants of 0–6 months unless circumstances prescribe otherwise.

A59 E

Gastro-oesophageal reflux in infants is common and tends to resolve at 12–18 months of age. Simple procedures, such as posture and thickening of foods, may help to alleviate gastro-oesophageal disease in infants.

A60 A

Clinical signs of dehydration in children include tachycardia, loss of skin turgor and dry tongue.

A61 B

Mumps is an acute viral infection transmitted by airborne droplets. Mumps is considered to be a childhood infection affecting those between 5 and 15 years of age. Classic symptoms of mumps include fever, chills, malaise, and enlargement of the parotid glands, which may be unilateral or bilateral. The swelling of the parotid glands may result in the patient experiencing a dry mouth because saliva flow is blocked.

A62 C

Characteristic symptoms of allergic rhinitis (hay fever) include itchy nose, prolonged sneezing attacks, rhinorrhoea and red, itchy eyes (conjunctival lacrimation).

A63 E

Cataracts refer to the opacity of the lens of the eye or of its capsule. Symptoms of cataracts are a progressive decrease in visual acuity as the lens becomes visibly opaque. Cataracts are usually painless but pain may be an accompanying symptom if the cataract swells and secondary glaucoma develops.

A64 C

Calcipotriol is a vitamin D derivative used topically for psoriasis. It does not cause skin discoloration and does not stain clothes.

A65   B

Ciclosporin is a potent immunosuppressant, which is markedly nephrotoxic. It may cause gastrointestinal disturbances. Ciclosporin is available as capsules, oral solution and parenteral preparations.

A66   A

As with other quinolones, ciprofloxacin should be used with caution in epileptic patients, in children, during pregnancy and breast-feeding.

A67   A

Arthrotec tablets contain the non-steroidal anti-inflammatory drug diclofenac and the prostaglandin misoprostol. The combination of the two active ingredients makes Arthrotec suitable in patients predisposed to gastrointestinal ulceration. Dulcolax (bisacodyl) tablets act as a stimulant laxative. Voltarol Retard tablets contain the non-steroidal anti-inflammatory drug diclofenac. All three preparations must be swallowed whole without being chewed.

A68   E

Ranitidine is a H_2-receptor antagonist, which reduces the gastric output. Unlike cimetidine, ranitidine does not interact with cytochrome P450, so does not retard hepatic metabolism of certain drugs, such as warfarin. Ranitidine may be administered as 150 mg twice daily or 300 mg at night.

A69   C

Both omeprazole, a proton pump inhibitor and paclitaxel, a taxane cytotoxic may cause nausea and vomiting as side-effects. Prednisolone, as with other corticosteroids, does not cause nausea and vomiting. Corticosteroids such as dexamethasone are administered to relieve nausea and vomiting particularly that associated with chemotherapy.

A70   A

Levodopa is the amino precursor of dopamine. It is used to replenish depleted dopamine in Parkinson's disease. Levodopa may cause insomnia, reddish discoloration of urine and headache.

A71   B

Levocobastine is used in the treatment of allergic rhinitis (hay fever) and allergic conjunctivitis. It is available as an aqueous nasal spray and can be applied as two sprays into each nostril twice daily, increased if necessary to four times daily.

A72   B

Headaches that are constantly painful and seem to be particularly worse in the morning may be associated with uncontrolled hypertension. Patients presenting with headaches accompanied by fever and neck stiffness should be referred.

A73   C

Periodontitis is a dental condition caused by bacteria where plaque-induced inflammatory changes affect the periodontal ligament and the alveolar bone leading to loss of the periodontal structure and resorption of the alveolar bone. Periodontitis which, unlike gingivitis, is not reversible, tends to be chronic and requires referral.

A74 C

Cystitis is a urinary tract bacterial infection generally caused by *Escherichia coli*. It results in inflammation of the bladder and urethra and is characterised by a frequent urge to pass urine accompanied by a burning or stinging sensation on urination. Cystitis is common in females but less common in men who must always be referred. Children are always referred as urinary tract infections make children susceptible to permanent kidney and bladder damage. Management of cystitis is based on the administration of alkalinising agents to help restore the pH of the urine to normal non-acidic environment. The alkalinising agents are administered three times daily for two days and the risk of hyperkalaemia is negligible.

A75 C

Tamoxifen is an oestrogen-receptor antagonist indicated as adjuvant hormonal treatment in oestrogen-receptor-positive breast cancer in post-menopausal women. Common side-effects include alopecia and uterine fibroids.

A76 E

In nicotine replacement therapy, the chewing gum releases nicotine which is absorbed through the buccal mucosa every time a piece of chewing gum is chewed. The chewing gum is chewed for 30 minutes, only when one feels the urge to smoke. The transdermal patch provides a residual nicotine level throughout the application. A side-effect of nicotine chewing gum may be aphthous ulcers.

A77 E

Zolpidem is an imidazopyridine but not a benzodiazepine; however, it acts on the same receptors as benzodiazepines. Zolpidem has a short duration of action and is indicated for patients who have difficulty sleeping. It does not have any hangover effects. The dose of Zolpidem should be reduced in patients with hepatic impairment and it should be avoided in cases of severe hepatic impairment.

A78 E

Orciprenaline is a partially selective adrenoceptor-agonist and hence it is more likely to have effects on the cardiovascular system, such as arrhythmias, than the selective adrenoceptor-agonists, such as salbutamol, terbutaline and the long-acting beta-agonists salmeterol and formoterol. Orciprenaline is available only as tablets or syrup and can be prescribed to 4-year-old children.

A79 C

Gliclazide is a sulphonylurea. Gliclazide has a short half-life, unlike gliben-clamide. For this reason elderly patients are often given gliclazide, to avoid hypoglycaemic attacks, which are more often associated with long-acting sulphonylureas. Fluconazole (triazole antifungal) interacts with the sulphonyl-ureas by increasing the plasma concentration of sulphonylureas when both drugs are administered concomitantly.

A80 E

Typhoid fever is caused by *Salmonella typhii* bacilli. The condition has an incu-bation period of about 5–23 days. Classic symptoms of typhoid fever include headache, abdominal pain with constipation or diarrhoea. Rose-coloured spots and macular rashes on the abdomen are characteristic of typhoid fever.

A81 B

Largactil is a proprietary preparation of chlorpromazine, an aliphatic antipsy-chotic with marked sedation and moderate antimuscarinic and extrapyramidal side-effects. Serenace is a proprietary preparation of haloperidol, a butyro-phenone antipsychotic with marked extrapyramidal side-effects, moderate sedation but not very likely to cause hypotension. Tegretol is a proprietary preparation of carbamazepine, an anti-epileptic drug indicated in simple and complex partial seizures and for tonic-clonic seizures.

A82   D

Prophylaxis for malaria includes the administration of antimalarial tablets and protection against mosquito bites but does not include any vaccinations. Hepatitis C is a viral infection and no vaccine is available. Hepatitis B is a viral infection and prophylaxis is provided by a vaccine.

A83   B

Griseofulvin and terbinafine are indicated in the management of fungal nail infections. Nystatin (polyene antifungal) is indicated in the management of *Candida* infections and is not indicated for fungal nail infections.

A84   C

Orlistat is a pancreatic lipase inhibitor used in conjunction with a hypocaloric diet to reduce the absorption of dietary fat in obese patients. Orlistat is administered twice daily immediately before, during or up to 1 hour after each meal. If the meal contains no fat there is no need to take Orlistat.

A85   A

All angiotensin-converting enzyme inhibitors including enalapril, may precipitate a hypoglycaemic attack in a diabetic patient because enalapril may potentiate the effect of sulphonylureas.

A86   E

Repaglinide is a newer oral hypoglycaemic agent, indicated in type 2 diabetes either in combination with metformin or as monotherapy. Repaglinide stimulates insulin release.

A87   E

Urinalysis for glucose monitoring can detect hyperglycaemia but not hypoglycaemia. Blood glucose monitoring gives a direct measure of the glucose concentration at the time of the test. It can detect both hyperglycaemia and hypoglycaemia and it is used in preference to urinalysis. Random blood glucose concentrations must be maintained at <7.8 mmol/L (140 mg/dL).

A88   D

Both budesonide and fluticasone are corticosteroids but fluticasone is more potent than budesonide and has a higher first-pass effect, hence more of the drug is metabolised leading to fewer adverse effects. A dose of 100 μg of budesonide is equivalent to 50 μg of fluticasone. Both budesonide and fluticasone are indicated for the prophylaxis of allergic rhinitis (hay fever).

A89   B

Xalatan drops is a proprietary preparation of latanoprost (prostaglandin analogue), indicated in glaucoma.

A90   A

Xalatan (latanoprost) is a prostaglandin analogue, which increases the uvoscleral outflow, thereby decreasing the intra-ocular pressure. The drops, which are applied once daily, preferably in the evening, may cause eye discoloration especially in patients with mixed colour irides.

A91 C

Benzamycin gel is a proprietary preparation and contains benzoyl peroxide and erythromycin (macrolide antibiotic).

A92 D

Benzamycin may cause redness of the skin, in which case the treatment is stopped and re-introduced at a reduced frequency.

A93 C

Benzamycin is indicated in patients with acne.

A94 D

Benzamycin is available as gel, which must be reconstituted by the pharmacist prior to dispensing. The patient should be advised to avoid excessive exposure to sunlight.

A95 B

Zestril contains lisinopril, an angiotensin-converting enzyme inhibitor. Angiotensin-converting enzyme inhibitors tend to retain potassium, thereby counteracting the potassium loss caused by the thiazide diuretic bendro-flumethiazide (bendrofluazide).

A96 C

Concomitant administration of methotrexate and Voltarol, a proprietary preparation of diclofenac, a non-steroidal anti-inflammatory drug, may result in accumulation of methotrexate as its excretion is reduced. The use of diclofenac and diuretics such as bendroflumethiazide (bendrofluazide) may increase the risk of nephrotoxicity. Concomitant use of alcohol and an angiotensin-converting enzyme inhibitor such as lisinopril (Zestril) may result in an enhanced hypotensive effect. Alcohol and the benzodiazepine diazepam (Valium) may result in enhanced sedation.

A97 D

Methotrexate is a cytotoxic agent which may cause pulmonary toxicity and therefore patients are advised to contact the doctor if cough develops.

A98 A

Methotrexate is an antimetabolite, which is metabolised by the renal and hepatic systems and may lead to renal and hepatic toxicities. Liver and renal function tests are therefore carried out for patients who are administered the drug. Methotrexate can lead to myelosuppression and therefore full blood counts must be monitored for patients taking it.

A99 D

Methotrexate is one of the disease-modifying antirheumatic drugs, which are administered once a week. The initial dose is 7.5 mg administered once a week and the maximum dose is 15–20 mg administered once a week.

A100 A

Deltacortil is a proprietary preparation of the corticosteroid prednisolone. As with other corticosteroids, prednisolone may lead to precipitation of osteoporosis, insomnia and candidiasis.

Test 3

Questions

Questions 1–22

Directions: Each of the questions or incomplete statements is followed by five suggested answers. Select the best answer in each case.

Q1 The refrigerator in the pharmacy that is used for storage of pharmaceutical products should be kept at a temperature of:

A ☐ 0–3 °C
B ☐ 2–8 °C
C ☐ 5–10 °C
D ☐ 6–12 °C
E ☐ –3–8 °C

Q2 A patient with diverticular disease is instructed to take a laxative. The pharmacist should appropriately recommend:

A ☐ Senokot tablets
B ☐ Dulcolax tablets
C ☐ glycerol suppositories
D ☐ Fybogel sachets
E ☐ Milk of Magnesia suspension

Q3 A patient comes into the pharmacy with rhinorrhoea. Which of the following list of symptoms is most likely to indicate allergic rhinitis?

A ☐ coloured sputum
B ☐ fever

C ☐ sore throat

D ☐ sneezing

E ☐ malaise

Q4 What is the dose of mefenamic acid that can be given to a child of 3 years, considering that the dosing regimen is 25 mg/kg daily in divided doses?

A ☐ 10 mL t.d.s.

B ☐ 5 mL t.d.s.

C ☐ 2.5 mL t.d.s.

D ☐ 5 mL b.d.

E ☐ 7 mL t.d.s.

Q5 Which of the following products could be responsible for causing constipation?

A ☐ Ponstyl

B ☐ Adalat

C ☐ Codipront

D ☐ Amoxil

E ☐ Dulcolax

Q6 Over-the-counter products which may be recommended to prevent napkin dermatitis include all EXCEPT:

A ☐ zinc and castor oil ointment

B ☐ Vasogen

C ☐ Sudocrem

D ☐ Travocort

E ☐ Conotrane

Q7   A physician calls the pharmacist and enquires about a sustained release NSAID for a patient who has sciatica. Of the following products, the pharmacist could suggest:

A   ☐ Nu-seals tablets
B   ☐ Contac 400 capsules
C   ☐ Distalgesic tablets
D   ☐ Oruvail capsules
E   ☐ Tramal tablets

Q8   A patient comes to the pharmacy complaining of sore, tired eyes. Which drug would you recommend over-the-counter?

A   ☐ tropicamide
B   ☐ naphazoline
C   ☐ hypromellose
D   ☐ betamethasone
E   ☐ timolol maleate

Q9   When comparing amlodipine and nifedipine, amlodipine:

A   ☐ has a longer duration of action
B   ☐ can be used in hypertension
C   ☐ is available as a spray formulation
D   ☐ causes ankle swelling as a side-effect
E   ☐ cannot be used in angina

Q10   A micro-organism that is associated with serious complications if associated with eye infections is:

A   ☐ herpes simplex virus
B   ☐ *Escherichia coli*

C   ☐ *Pseudomonas aeruginosa*
D   ☐ *Aspergillus niger*
E   ☐ *Bacillus subtilis*

Q11   Gingivitis refers to inflammation of the:

A   ☐ pharynx
B   ☐ tongue
C   ☐ gums
D   ☐ larynx
E   ☐ salivary gland

Q12   Which of the following is NOT an inflammatory mediator?

A   ☐ bradykinin
B   ☐ histamine
C   ☐ lymphokines
D   ☐ glucose
E   ☐ lysosomal enzymes

Q13   Otitis media is caused by the following micro-organisms EXCEPT:

A   ☐ *Staphylococcus aureus*
B   ☐ *Haemophilus influenzae*
C   ☐ *Streptococcus pyogenes*
D   ☐ *Pseudomonas aeruginosa*
E   ☐ *Enterobius vermicularis*

Q14   A patient comes to the pharmacy requesting Solpadeine capsules, which are currently out-of-stock. Which product would you recommend as a substitute?

A ☐ Anadin

B ☐ Night Nurse

C ☐ Syndol

D ☐ Codis

E ☐ Dristan

Q15 Which of the following drugs is associated with precipitation of a migraine attack?

A ☐ aspirin

B ☐ combined oral contraceptives

C ☐ metoclopramide

D ☐ propranolol

E ☐ diazepam

Q16 Which of the following is NOT a cytotoxic drug?

A ☐ vincristine

B ☐ fluorouracil

C ☐ ciclosporin

D ☐ bleomycin

E ☐ methotrexate

Q17 Legionnaire's disease affects primarily the:

A ☐ respiratory system

B ☐ urinary tract

C ☐ skin

D ☐ eye

E ☐ gums

Q18   Gingival hyperplasia is associated with:

A   ☐ digoxin
B   ☐ phenytoin
C   ☐ enalapril
D   ☐ theophylline
E   ☐ captopril

Q19   A patient asks for Actifed tablets, which is currently not available at the pharmacy. What alternative product can be dispensed?

A   ☐ Mucosolvan syrup
B   ☐ Rhinopront capsules
C   ☐ Uniflu tablets
D   ☐ Meggezones lozenges
E   ☐ Codipront capsules

Q20   Appropriate preparations that could be dispensed over-the-counter for athlete's foot include all of the following EXCEPT:

A   ☐ Systral cream
B   ☐ Canesten cream
C   ☐ Scholl Athlete's foot cream
D   ☐ Daktarin powder
E   ☐ Scholl Athlete's foot spray

Q21   A patient comes to the pharmacy with multiple mosquito bites. Which of the following preparations would be most suitable?

A   ☐ paracetamol tablets
B   ☐ hydrocortisone cream
C   ☐ fusidic acid cream

D ☐ benzocaine spray

E ☐ mepyramine cream

Q22 The molecular structure of ampicillin is shown below.

This structure may be modified to produce amoxicillin by attaching a (an):

A ☐ hydroxyl group

B ☐ amide

C ☐ aldehyde

D ☐ hydroxyl group and carboxylic group

E ☐ hydroxyl group and chloride group

Questions 23–40

Directions: Each group of questions below consists of five lettered headings followed by a list of numbered questions. For each numbered question select the one heading that is most closely related to it. Each heading may be used once, more than once, or not at all.

Questions 23–26 concern the following antacid preparations:

A ☐ Rennie tablets

B ☐ Maalox suspension

C ☐ Setlers Wind-eze

D ☐ Milk of Magnesia suspension

E ☐ Sodium bicarbonate powder

Select, from A to E, which one of the above:

Q23   is most suitable for treating abdominal discomfort caused by trapped gas

Q24   is most suitable for a patient requesting immediate relief from dyspepsia

Q25   is most suitable for a patient suffering chronically from heartburn

Q26   is most suitable for a pregnant woman whose gynaecologist suggested an antacid

Questions 27–29 concern the following vitamin and mineral supplements:

A   ☐ Forceval
B   ☐ Arcalion
C   ☐ Fefol
D   ☐ Ca-C
E   ☐ Selenium-ACE

Select, from A to E, which one of the above:

Q27   is suitable for a patient who requests a multivitamin preparation

Q28   is suitable for iron and folic acid supplementation during pregnancy

Q29   is suitable for a 50-year-old woman as a calcium supplement

Questions 30–32 concern the following haemorrhoidal preparations:

A   ☐ Proctosedyl
B   ☐ Preparation H
C   ☐ Soframycin
D   ☐ Anusol
E   ☐ Nupercainal

Select, from A to E, which one of the above:

Q30 is suitable for a patient with haemorrhoids where inflammation is severe

Q31 is a preparation that contains a local anaesthetic only

Q32 contains astringents that are useful in the treatment of haemorrhoids

Questions 33–35 concern the following drugs:

A ☐ metoclopramide
B ☐ promethazine
C ☐ cinnarizine
D ☐ cyclizine
E ☐ hyoscine

Select, from A to E, which one of the above:

Q33 is ineffective in motion sickness

Q34 can be recommended for motion sickness when a sedative effect is desired

Q35 acts on the chemoreceptor trigger zone

Questions 36–40 concern the following cautionary labels:

A ☐ 'May cause drowsiness. If affected do not drive or operate machinery'
B ☐ 'Swallowed whole, not chewed'
C ☐ 'Avoid exposure of skin to direct sunlight or sunlamps'
D ☐ 'Avoid alcoholic drink'
E ☐ 'Take an hour before food or on an empty stomach'

Select, from A to E, which one of the above should be used when dispensing:

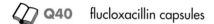 **Q36**   Dulcolax tablets

Q37   Slow-K tablets

Q38   Zaditen syrup

Q39   Euglucon tablets

Q40   flucloxacillin capsules

Questions 41–84

Directions: For each of the questions below, ONE or MORE of the responses is (are) correct. Decide which of the responses is (are) correct. Then choose:

A   ☐ if 1, 2 and 3 are correct
B   ☐ if 1 and 2 only are correct
C   ☐ if 2 and 3 only are correct
D   ☐ if 1 only is correct
E   ☐ if 3 only is correct

Directions summarised				
A	**B**	**C**	**D**	**E**
1, 2, 3	1, 2 only	2, 3 only	1 only	3 only

Q41 Care should be taken with the use of the following drugs in a patient with hepatic impairment:

1 ☐ statins
2 ☐ antihistamines
3 ☐ selective serotonin re-uptake inhibitors

Q42 Drugs that can significantly interact adversely with calcium-channel blockers include:

1 ☐ atenolol
2 ☐ ranitidine
3 ☐ enalapril

Q43 Products that should be stored in a refrigerator include:

1 ☐ ACT-HIB
2 ☐ Daktacort cream
3 ☐ Garamycin eye drops

Q44 A patient with hypertension (male 56 years, weight 55 kg) visits the pharmacy with a new prescription for nabumetone. The patient is already taking enalapril 20 mg daily, atenolol 100 mg daily and bendroflumethiazide (bendrofluazide) 2.5 mg daily. Which of the following statement(s) is (are) true?

1 ☐ the patient may experience a hypotensive reaction
2 ☐ the patient may experience a hypertensive reaction
3 ☐ there is an increased risk of nephrotoxicity

Q45 Which of the following drug combinations would be queried with the prescriber as causing potentially clinically significant interactions?

1 ☐ propranolol and nifedipine
2 ☐ amitriptyline and co-amoxiclav
3 ☐ carbamazepine and cefuroxime axetil

Q46   When testing body fluids in a pharmacy, it is recommended that:

1   ☐ tests are carried out in a designated area in the pharmacy
2   ☐ contaminated waste is disposed of in an appropriate dustbin
3   ☐ test is undertaken after opening hours

Q47   Which of the following statement(s) is (are) correct about omeprazole?

1   ☐ it inhibits gastric acid by blocking the hydrogen-potassium adenosine triphosphate enzyme system of the gastric parietal cell
2   ☐ side-effects expected include diarrhoea, headache, nausea and vomiting
3   ☐ concomitant use with phenytoin is associated with enhanced effects of phenytoin

Q48   Which of the following statement(s) is (are) true about digoxin?

1   ☐ it has a long half-life
2   ☐ side-effects include nausea, vomiting, diarrhoea, abdominal pain, arrhythmias
3   ☐ a geriatric dosage formulation is available as 0.0625 mg tablets

Q49   Patients taking amiodarone should be advised to:

1   ☐ avoid exposure to sunlight
2   ☐ use a sun protection lotion daily
3   ☐ be careful when driving at night

Q50   When dispensing simvastatin, the patient should be advised to:

1   ☐ report promptly unexplained muscle pain, tenderness and weakness
2   ☐ take dose at night
3   ☐ follow dietary measures

Q51 Sumatriptan should be used with caution in patients:

1 ☐ with a history of angina
2 ☐ taking fluoxetine
3 ☐ taking enalapril maleate

Q52 Doxycycline:

1 ☐ is contraindicated in children under 12 years
2 ☐ cannot be used in patients with kidney disease
3 ☐ is only active against Gram-positive organisms

Q53 Which of the following drugs should be avoided in breast-feeding?

1 ☐ aspirin
2 ☐ diazepam
3 ☐ amoxicillin

Q54 Referral is warranted when a patient presents with a headache that is:

1 ☐ accompanied by nausea, vomiting and nose bleeds
2 ☐ accompanied by paraesthesia, numbness
3 ☐ unilateral

Q55 Croup:

1 ☐ occurs in young children
2 ☐ is characterised by a barking cough
3 ☐ may lead to cyanosis and respiratory failure

Q56 Verrucas:

1 ☐ are caused by the human papilloma virus
2 ☐ are characterised by a cauliflower-like appearance
3 ☐ may be contracted in swimming pools and public baths

Q57 Hiatus hernia:

1 ☐ is the protrusion of a portion of the stomach into the thorax
2 ☐ may be asymptomatic
3 ☐ is common in obese patients

Q58 Gluten-free products are recommended to patients with:

1 ☐ coeliac disease
2 ☐ diabetes mellitus
3 ☐ liver disease

Q59 Chilblains:

1 ☐ are local inflammatory lesions
2 ☐ occur in cold conditions
3 ☐ are accompanied by intense pruritus

Q60 Migraine headache:

1 ☐ may be precipitated by ingestion of chocolate
2 ☐ may be preceded by an aura
3 ☐ is due to sustained contraction of skeletal muscle

Q61 Stemetil:

1 ☐ is used for labyrinthine disorders
2 ☐ should be used with caution with paracetamol
3 ☐ is available only as a parenteral dosage formulation

Q62 Septicaemia:

1 ☐ occurs when pathogenic micro-organisms are present in the blood
2 ☐ is characterised by fever, chills, diarrhoea, nausea and vomiting
3 ☐ is caused only by fungi

Q63 Hypokalaemia:

1   ☐ is characterised by plasma potassium concentration below 60 mmol/l
2   ☐ may be caused by diuretic therapy
3   ☐ is characterised by muscle weakness, cramps

Q64 Patients who complain of abdominal pain should be referred when:

1   ☐ they describe pain as unbearable
2   ☐ it is associated with rapid weight loss
3   ☐ accompanying symptoms include vomiting and constipation

Q65 Infantile seborrhoeic dermatitis:

1   ☐ is one type of eczema
2   ☐ may be relieved by rubbing almond oil before washing the hair
3   ☐ is due to an infection by a micro-organism

Q66 Lithium:

1   ☐ is used in the prophylaxis of mania
2   ☐ has a narrow therapeutic index
3   ☐ cannot be used concurrently with diuretics

Q67 Knee caps:

1   ☐ are indicated for soft tissue support
2   ☐ are contraindicated in patients taking NSAIDS
3   ☐ may cause hypersensitivity reactions

Q68   Preparations that could be recommended to a patient who is complaining of dry skin include:

1   ☐ E45 cream
2   ☐ Oilatum bath additive
3   ☐ Solarcaine gel

Q69   Products used for ear wax removal include:

1   ☐ Cerumol
2   ☐ Waxsol
3   ☐ Locorten-Vioform

Q70   Drugs that may have an adverse effect on contact lens wear include:

1   ☐ Phenergan
2   ☐ Valium
3   ☐ Logynon

Q71   Which of the following drugs do NOT cause dependence?

1   ☐ zolmitriptan
2   ☐ pethidine
3   ☐ morphine

Q72   Neural tube defects are associated with administration during pregnancy of:

1   ☐ phenytoin
2   ☐ carbamazepine
3   ☐ valproate

Q73 A patient comes to the pharmacy requesting Vermox tablets. What advice should be given?

1 ☐ dosage regimen is four times daily for 5 days
2 ☐ Vermox can be used in children under 1 year
3 ☐ all the members of the family should be treated

Q74 A patient comes to the pharmacy requesting advice on a cold. Which of the following symptoms would indicate referral?

1 ☐ rhinorrhoea
2 ☐ dysphagia
3 ☐ pain on coughing

Q75 Beechams Hot Lemon and Honey should be avoided in patients with:

1 ☐ glaucoma
2 ☐ hypertension
3 ☐ diabetes mellitus

Q76 The laxative action of Duphalac results from:

1 ☐ osmosis
2 ☐ increase in synthesis of prostaglandins
3 ☐ support of growth of colonic bacteria

Q77 Drugs which have a narrow therapeutic index include:

1 ☐ phenytoin
2 ☐ theophylline
3 ☐ codeine

Q78 The advantages of selective serotonin re-uptake inhibitors over the tricyclic antidepressants include:

1. ☐ lower incidence of antimuscarinic side-effects
2. ☐ better effectiveness
3. ☐ less likely to cause gastrointestinal side-effects

Q79 A woman comes to the pharmacy with severe sunburn. Which of the following should be advised?

1. ☐ apply a soothing antiseptic cream
2. ☐ drink plenty of water
3. ☐ apply local anaesthetic

Q80 Dandruff:

1. ☐ is a form of seborrhoeic dermatitis
2. ☐ may indicate the use of Betnovate lotion
3. ☐ suggests the recommendation of shampoos containing coal tar

Q81 Calamine lotion:

1. ☐ has a cooling effect
2. ☐ may be used for chickenpox to promote skin healing
3. ☐ has an emollient effect

Q82 Side-effects that may result in a patient taking 50 mg prednisolone daily for 3 months include:

1. ☐ peptic ulceration
2. ☐ adrenal suppression
3. ☐ subcapsular cataracts

Q83 Sibutramine:

1. ☐ is an opioid drug
2. ☐ inhibits re-uptake of noradrenaline (norepinephrine) and serotonin
3. ☐ is a centrally acting appetite suppressant

Q84   Back pain may be associated with:

1   ☐ otitis media
2   ☐ osteoporosis
3   ☐ pregnancy

Questions 85–91

Directions: The following questions consist of a first statement followed by a second statement. Decide whether the first statement is true or false. Decide whether the second statement is true or false. Then choose:

A   ☐ if both statements are true and the second statement is a *correct explanation* of the first statement

B   ☐ if both statements are true but the second statement *is NOT a correct explanation* of the first statement

C   ☐ if the first statement is true but the second statement is false

D   ☐ if the first statement is false but the second statement is true

E   ☐ if both statements are false

Directions summarised			
	First statement	**Second statement**	
A	True	True	Second statement is a *correct explanation* of the first
B	True	True	Second statement is *NOT a correct explanation* of the first
C	True	False	
D	False	True	
E	False	False	

Q85 Patients taking Uniflu (two every 4 h when required) should be advised not to take any remedies containing paracetamol. The maximum dose of paracetamol is 6 g in 24 h.

Q86 Dequacaine lozenges should be recommended to a patient who is diabetic. Dequacaine contain dequalinium chloride and benzocaine.

Q87 The use of Buscopan tablets is contraindicated in angle closure glaucoma. Buscopan is a quaternary ammonium compound.

Q88 Bactroban is available as a topical ointment. Bactroban is effective for skin infections caused by Gram-positive organisms.

Q89 Patients taking warfarin should be cautioned not to take medication containing aspirin. Aspirin can cause gastrointestinal bleeding.

Q90 Digital thermometers are safer to use in children than glass thermometers. Digital thermometers are cheaper than glass thermometers.

Q91 Lower initial doses of diuretics should be used in the elderly. The elderly are particularly susceptible to postural hypotension.

Questions 92–100

Directions: These questions involve cases. Read the prescription or case and answer the questions.

Questions 92–93: Use the prescription below:

Patient's name ....

Tinaderm: Otosporin 1 : 1
Apply 2 drops t.d.s. in each ear

Doctor's signature ....

Q92 When dispensing the product the following should be included on the label:

1   ☐ expiration date within 4 weeks of dispensing
2   ☐ expiration date within 2 days of dispensing
3   ☐ keep refrigerated

A   ☐ 1, 2, 3
B   ☐ 1, 2 only
C   ☐ 2, 3 only
D   ☐ 1 only
E   ☐ 3 only

Q93 The preparation is prescribed when the patient has:

A   ☐ otitis externa
B   ☐ otitis interna
C   ☐ otitis media
D   ☐ tinnitus
E   ☐ impacted cerumen

Question 94–96: Use the patient profile below:

Patient medication file

Patient's name ....

Age   59 years

Allergies   none

Diagnosis   hypertension

Medication record   atenolol 100 mg om
                    enalapril maleate 20 mg on
                    bendroflumethiazide (bendrofluazide) 5 mg o.m.

The patient comes to the pharmacy complaining of a sudden onset of severe pain in his foot. When the pharmacist examines the patient's foot, the great toe is red and swollen.

Q94   What condition is the patient likely to have?

A   ☐ strain
B   ☐ sprain
C   ☐ arthritis
D   ☐ sting
E   ☐ gout

Q95   Which drug is most likely to be the causative agent of the condition?

1   ☐ bendroflumethiazide (bendrofluazide)
2   ☐ bendroflumethiazide (bendrofluazide) and enalapril
3   ☐ atenolol

A   ☐ 1, 2, 3
B   ☐ 1, 2 only
C   ☐ 2, 3 only
D   ☐ 1 only
E   ☐ 3 only

Q96   Treatment of the condition may be addressed using:

A   ☐ NSAIDs
B   ☐ RICE (rest, ice, compression, elevation) regime
C   ☐ opioid analgesics
D   ☐ corticosteroids
E   ☐ calcitonin

Questions 97–100: Use the prescription below:

Patient's name   ....
24 years
Ciprofloxacin 250 mg
b.d.   m. 10
Doctor's signature   ....

Q97   Which product would you dispense when this prescription is presented?

A   ☐ Mictral
B   ☐ Cymalon
C   ☐ Ciprobay
D   ☐ Distaclor
E   ☐ Noroxin

Q98   The patient informs the pharmacist that the physician prescribed the medicine for a urinary tract infection. What non-pharmaceutical advice would you give the patient?

1   ☐ avoid intake of high-fibre foods
2   ☐ increase alcohol intake
3   ☐ increase fluid intake

A   ☐ 1, 2, 3
B   ☐ 1, 2 only
C   ☐ 2, 3 only
D   ☐ 1 only
E   ☐ 3 only

Q99 Ciprofloxacin:

1 ☐ is active against Gram-positive and Gram-negative bacteria
2 ☐ should be used with caution in patients taking NSAIDs
3 ☐ may cause nausea, vomiting, and dyspepsia as side-effects

A ☐ 1, 2, 3
B ☐ 1, 2 only
C ☐ 2, 3 only
D ☐ 1 only
E ☐ 3 only

Q100 Urinary tract infections are most commonly caused by:

A ☐ *Helicobacter pylori*
B ☐ *Campylobacter jejuni*
C ☐ *Escherichia coli*
D ☐ *Mycobacterium tuberculosis*
E ☐ rhinovirus

Test 3

Answers

A1 B

The refrigerator in the pharmacy intended for the storage of pharmaceutical items should be kept at a temperature of between 2° and 8 °C.

A2 D

Fybogel sachets contain ispaghula husk, a bulk-forming laxative, which relieves constipation by increasing the faecal mass through peristalsis. Bulk-forming laxatives are indicated to alleviate constipation in patients with diverticular disease and they could be used on a long-term basis. Patients are also advised to maintain an adequate fluid intake and a diet rich in fibre. Senokot tablets (sennosides), Dulcolax tablets (bisacodyl) and glycerol suppositories are classified as stimulant laxatives. These increase intestinal motility and must be avoided in intestinal obstruction, such as may occur in diverticular disease. Milk of Magnesia (magnesium hydroxide), which is an osmotic laxative is not indicated in diverticular disease.

A3 D

Sneezing, together with a runny or congested nose and red, itchy eyes, is the most common feature of allergic rhinitis (hay fever). Coloured sputum, fever, sore throat and malaise indicate the presence of an infection, rather than an allergic component.

A4 A

A 3-year-old child weighs approximately 15 kg. The daily dosing regimen for this patient would be:

25 mg × 15 kg = 375 mg

Mefenamic acid suspension is available as 50 mg/5 mL.

The patient therefore must be given 37.5 mL to receive the total daily dose of 375 mg; 37.5 mL divided into three doses in a day would be equivalent to 12.5 mL. This means that the patient must be given 10 mL on a three times daily (t.d.s.) basis.

A5   C

Codipront contains the opioid antitussive codeine and the antihistamine phenyltoloxamine. One of the side-effects of opioids is constipation. Ponstyl is a proprietary (trade name) preparation of the non-steroidal anti-inflammatory drug mefenamic acid; Adalat is a proprietary preparation of the calcium-channel blocker nifedipine; Amoxil is a proprietary preparation of the beta-lactam amoxicillin; and Dulcolax is the brand name of the stimulant laxative bisacodyl.

A6   D

Napkin dermatitis can be soothed and prevented with the use of barrier creams and ointments such as zinc and castor oil, Vasogen, Sudocrem and Conotrane. Travocort contains an antifungal isoconazole nitrate and the potent corticosteroid difluocortolone. Such combination products are only indicated in severe napkin dermatitis and are used only for one week after which treatment is continued with a cream containing an antifungal only.

A7   D

Oruvail is a brand-name preparation available as sustained release capsules containing the non-steroidal anti-inflammatory drug ketoprofen. Nu-seals is a proprietary preparation of enteric-coated aspirin 75 mg; Contac 400 is the trade name for the cold preparation containing the nasal decongestant phenylpropanolamine and the antihistamine chlorphenamine (chlorpheniramine). Distalgesic is a proprietary preparation of the analgesic combination co-proxamol, containing paracetamol and the mild opioid analgesic dextropropoxyphene. Tramal is a trade-marked product containing the opioid analgesic tramadol.

A8   B

Naphazoline is a sympathomimetic decongestant that is soothing in sore, tired eyes. Tropicamide is a short-acting antimuscarinic, which dilates the pupil and is therefore administered before eye examinations. Hypromellose is indicated in dry eyes. Betamethasone is a corticosteroid preparation, the use of which as an ophthalmic preparation is usually avoided as administration of corticosteroids to the eye may exacerbate unconfirmed herpes simplex viral infections, cause steroid glaucoma or steroid cataract. Timolol maleate is a beta-blocker used in glaucoma.

A9   A

Amlodipine and nifedipine are dihydropyridine calcium-channel blockers. Amlodipine differs from nifedipine in that it has a longer duration of action and can therefore be given once daily, unlike nifedipine. Both are indicated in hypertension and angina and tend to cause ankle oedema which does not respond to diuretic therapy. Neither amlodipine nor nifedipine are available as spray formulations.

A10   C

Eye infections caused by *Pseudomonas aeruginosa* are associated with severe complications.

A11   C

Gingivitis refers to an inflammation of the gums, which may be caused by poor oral hygiene, dental defects, diabetes and mouth breathing. Gingivitis unlike periodontitis is reversible. Good oral hygiene is encouraged and patients are advised to use an antiseptic mouthwash regularly.

A12   D

Glucose is a simple sugar and is the sole provider of energy to the brain. It is stored in the body as glucagon. Bradykinin, histamine, lymphokines and lyso-somal enzymes are all different inflammatory mediators that play a significant role in precipitating asthma and other inflammatory conditions.

A13   E

Streptococcus aureus, *Haemophilus influenzae*, *Streptococcus pyogenes* and *Pseudomonas aeruginosa* are all micro-organisms that can cause otitis media. *Enterobius vermicularis* is a threadworm leading to an infection characterised by itchy anus and the presence of white worms.

A14   C

Solpadeine capsules contain paracetamol, the opioid analgesic codeine and the weak stimulant caffeine. Syndol is the other analgesic preparation com-bining paracetamol, codeine and caffeine. Syndol also contains the antihista-mine doxylamine. Anadin contains aspirin and caffeine. Night Nurse contains paracetamol, the antitussive dextromethorphan and the antihistamine prometh-azine. Codis contains aspirin and codeine. Dristan tablets contain aspirin, caffeine, the antihistamine chlorphenamine (chlorpheniramine) and the nasal decongestant phenylephrine.

A15   B

Combined oral contraceptives may cause migraine and are contraindicated in such patients. Progesterone-only contraceptives are more suitable in this case.

A16   C

Ciclosporin, a calcineurin inhibitor, is a potent immunosuppressant useful in the prevention of rejection in organ transplants and grafting procedures.

Ciclosporin is markedly nephrotoxic. Vincristine is a vinca alkaloid cytotoxic agent; fluorouracil and methotrexate are both antimetabolite cytotoxic agents; and bleomycin is a cytotoxic antibiotic.

A17 A

Legionnaire's disease is an acute respiratory disease caused by the Gram-negative, aerobic, non-sporing bacillus *Legionella pneumophila*. The disease is transmitted through the inhalation of infected water droplets.

A18 B

Ginvigal hyperplasia is a side-effect commonly associated with phenytoin.

A19 B

Actifed is a preparation containing pseudoephedrine (nasal decongestant) and triprolidine (antihistamine). Rhinopront capsules are an alternative preparation containing carbinoxamine, an antihistamine and phenylephrine, a nasal decongestant. Mucosolvan syrup contains ambroxol, a mucolytic agent indicated in chesty cough. Uniflu is a cold remedy preparation containing paracetamol, the opioid analgesic codeine, the antihistamine diphenhydramine, the nasal decongestant phenylephrine, ascorbic acid and caffeine. Meggezones lozenges contain menthol and are indicated in sore throats. Codipront capsules contain codeine as an antitussive and the antihistamine phenyltoloxamine.

A20 A

Systral cream is an antihistamine cream containing chlorphenoxamine. Athlete's foot is a fungal infection in which topical antifungal preparations are effective. Canesten cream contains clotrimazole, Daktarin powder contains miconazole and Scholl Athlete's foot preparations contain tolnaftate all indicated in the treatment of athlete's foot.

A21 B

The application of a mild topical corticosteroid, such as hydrocortisone, is effective in patients presenting with multiple mosquito bites. Paracetamol, which is an antipyretic agent is not indicated in mosquito bites. Fusidic acid cream is an anti-infective agent and is indicated if the mosquito bites have been scratched and there is risk of infection. Benzocaine (anaesthetic) and mepyramine (antihistamine) may relieve itchiness but are less effective in multiple mosquito bites than hydrocortisone.

A22 A

The difference between ampicillin and amoxicillin is the hydroxyl group that makes amoxicillin more soluble than ampicillin. Amoxicillin is in fact administered three times daily rather than four times daily.

A23 C

Setlers Wind-eze preparation contains activated dimeticone which is an antifoaming agent used to relieve flatulence and hence suitable for treating abdominal discomfort caused by trapped gas.

A24 A

Rennie tablets contain calcium carbonate and magnesium carbonate. Calcium carbonate has the greatest neutralising capacity of all antacids and is also long-acting. It is therefore useful in patients requesting immediate relief from heartburn.

A25 B

Maalox suspension contains aluminium hydroxide and magnesium hydroxide. The combination known as co-magaldrox is suitable for patients requiring antacids on a long-term basis. Magnesium hydroxide tends to act as a laxative but its effect is counteracted by aluminium hydroxide which is itself constipating. The combination is also long-acting as the two salts tend to be relatively insoluble in water.

A26 B

Sodium bicarbonate is contraindicated in pregnancy because it can lead to water retention and an increase in blood pressure. Calcium-containing antacids such as Rennie may precipitate hypercalcaemia. Activated dimeticone (Setlers Wind-eze) is not indicated as an antacid. Milk of Magnesia (magnesium hydroxide) suspension tends to act as a laxative and is therefore avoided in pregnancy. Maalox suspension (aluminium hydroxide, magnesium hydroxide) is the most safe to use in pregnancy because of the insolubility of the salts and the few side-effects.

A27 A

Forceval is a multivitamin preparation containing vitamins and minerals.

A28 C

Fefol contains iron (ferrous sulphate) and folic acid and is indicated during pregnancy.

A29 D

Ca-C is a calcium supplement preparation which may be used in a 50-year-old woman.

A30 A

Proctosedyl is a haemorrhoidal preparation containing cinchocaine (anaesthetic) and hydrocortisone (corticosteroid). Haemorrhoidal preparations containing corticosteroids are effective when the inflammation is severe.

A31 E

Nupercainal preparation contains only the anaesthetic cinchocaine.

A32 D

Anusol preparation contains bismuth oxide and zinc oxide which offers a mechanical protective barrier, whereas Peru balsam has some antiseptic properties. Astringents coagulate skin protein and mucus membranes thus forming a protective layer. They also reduce secretions from the damaged cells and therefore relieve local irritation and inflammation.

A33 A

Metoclopramide is ineffective in motion sickness as it acts selectively on the chemoreceptor trigger zone. Metoclopramide is effective in treating vomiting associated with gastroduodenal, biliary and hepatic disease, and postoperative vomiting.

A34 B

Promethazine is an antihistamine, which leads to sedation and is therefore used in motion sickness when a sedative effect is desired.

A35 A

Metoclopramide is a dopamine receptor antagonist, which acts selectively on the chemoreceptor trigger zone.

A36 B

Dulcolax tablets containing bisacodyl, a stimulant laxative, must be swallowed whole with water and not chewed to decrease occurrence of abdominal cramps.

A37 B

Slow-K is a modified-release preparation containing potassium chloride. Patients taking Slow-K are advised to take the tablets in an upright position, while standing or sitting. The tablets should be swallowed whole with plenty of water, to avoid gastrointestinal irritation.

A38 A

Zaditen syrup contains ketotifen, an antihistamine that may cause drowsiness. Patients are therefore advised not to drive or operate machinery.

A39 D

Euglucon is an oral hypoglycaemic agent containing glibenclamide, a sulpho-nylurea. All patients taking oral hypoglycaemic agents are advised to avoid alcohol as the combination of alcohol and oral hypoglycaemic agents may lead to hypoglycaemic attacks.

A40 E

Flucloxacillin is a penicillin that must be taken either an hour before food or on an empty stomach for better absorption.

A41 A

Statins should be avoided in active liver disease and unexplained raised serum transaminases. Some antihistamines, such as diphenhydramine and promethazine, should be used with caution in mild-to-moderate liver disease. Fluoxetine, like the other selective serotonin re-uptake inhibitors, must be avoided in hepatic impairment.

A42   D

Concurrent administration of beta-blockers, such as atenolol, and calcium-channel blockers may precipitate heart failure and bradycardia because of an additive effect.

A43   B

ACT-HIB is *Haemophilus influenzae* type B vaccine. All vaccines and Daktacort cream (miconazole and hydrocortisone) must be stored in the refrigerator at a temperature of between 2° and 8 °C.

A44   C

Nabumetone is a non-steroidal anti-inflammatory drug. NSAIDs interact with both angiotensin-converting enzyme inhibitors, such as enalapril, and beta-adrenoceptor blockers, such as propranolol, resulting in antagonism to the hypotensive reaction therefore leading to a hypertensive reaction. NSAIDs interact with diuretics, such as bendroflumethiazide (bendrofluazide), resulting in an increased risk of nephrotoxicity.

A45   D

Concurrent administration of beta-adrenoceptor blockers, such as propranolol, and calcium-channel blockers, such as nifedipine, should be avoided as the combination leads to precipitation of heart failure due to the additive bradycardia effect of the two agents.

A46   B

Diagnostic testing of body fluids must be carried out in a designated area in the pharmacy. Contaminated waste must be disposed in an appropriate dustbin.

A47   A

Omeprazole is classified as a proton pump inhibitor as it acts by blocking the hydrogen-potassium adenosine triphosphate enzyme system of the gastric parietal cells. Omeprazole therefore inhibits gastric acid release. Common side-effects associated with omeprazole include diarrhoea, headache, nausea and vomiting. Concurrent administration of omeprazole and phenytoin results in enhanced effects of phenytoin, which may lead to phenytoin toxicity.

A48   A

Digoxin is a potent positive inotropic cardiac glycoside. Digoxin has a long half-life which are usually administered once daily. Side-effects usually associated with overdose which are characteristic of digoxin toxicity include nausea, vomiting, abdominal pain, diarrhoea and arrhythmias. The geriatric digoxin formulation is available as 0.0625 mg (62.5 μg), marketed as Lanoxin tablets.

A49   A

Amiodarone is useful in the treatment of supraventricular and ventricular arrhythmias. Amiodarone tends to have a number of side-effects, such as photosensitivity. Patients are advised to avoid exposure to sunlight and apply a sun protection factor on a daily basis. Amiodarone may also cause reversible corneal microdeposits as a result of which patients find night glare irritating and so patients are advised to avoid driving at night.

A50   A

Simvastatin is a statin. Patients taking statins must be advised to immediately report any unexplained muscle pain, tenderness and weakness and to take the dose preferably at night. Patients must also be advised to follow dietary measures, namely avoid fatty foods and maintain a high-fibre diet.

A51   B

Sumatriptan is a $5HT_1$ (serotonin) agonist indicated in the treatment of migraine. Sumatriptan causes vasoconstriction and must therefore be used with caution in patients with coronary heart disease, such as angina. Concurrent administration of the agonist, sumatriptan and antagonists, such as fluoxetine, which is a selective serotonin re-uptake inhibitor, leads to increased CNS toxicity.

A52   D

Doxycycline, being a tetracycline, is contraindicated in children under 12 years and during pregnancy because tetracyclines tend to be deposited in growing bones and teeth, causing staining and dental hypoplasia. Doxycyline and minocycline are the only tetracyclines that do not exacerbate renal failure and may therefore be administered in patients with renal impairment. Tetracyclines are broad-spectrum antibiotics, active against Gram-negative and Gram-positive micro-organisms.

A53   B

Aspirin is avoided in breast-feeding because of the possibility of Reye's syndrome. Moreover if high doses of aspirin are used, the neonate may develop hypoprothrombinaemia. Benzodiazepines such as diazepam are present in milk and therefore should be avoided during breast-feeding. Amoxicillin can be safely administered during pregnancy and breast-feeding.

A54   B

Patients complaining of headache accompanied by nausea, vomiting, nose bleeds, paraesthesia and numbness should be referred.

A55   A

Croup is characterised by a barking cough with high-pitched wheezing that can be heard on expiration. The condition may be accompanied by fever, and tachypnoea. Croup is caused by oedema and inflammation of the larynx, epiglottis and vocal cords resulting in narrowing of the airway passages. Croup occurs in babies and young children. It usually occurs at night and may lead to cyanosis and respiratory failure. The condition is rare and requires referral.

A56   A

Verrucas are caused by the human papilloma virus. Verrucas are warts having a characteristic cauliflower-like appearance. Verrucas are contracted from swimming pools and public baths. They are painful when pressure is applied. Treatment involves removal of the hyperkeratolytic skin layers by the use of keratolytic agents such as salicylic acid.

A57   A

Hiatus hernia refers to the protrusion of a portion of the stomach into the thorax through the oesophageal hiatus of the diaphragm. Hiatus hernia is common in obese patients and during pregnancy. Very often the condition is asymptomatic.

A58   D

Coeliac disease refers to a chronic condition in which the small intestine has an unusual sensitivity to gluten. The condition may be secondary to lactose intolerance. Patients with coeliac disease must therefore follow a gluten-free diet.

A59   A

Chilblains are areas of the skin that are locally inflamed and bluish-red in colour. They occur as a reaction to cold, damp weather. The lesions are very often accompanied by tenderness and intense pruritus.

A60   B

Migraine headache may be triggered by a variety of factors, including chocolate. Patients are advised to try and identify triggering factors, to avoid migraine attacks as much as possible. Migraine attacks may or may not be preceded by an aura consisting of visual disturbances, blind spots or flashing lights. The aetiology of migraine is unknown. Sustained contraction of the skeletal muscle is associated with tension headache and not with migraine headache.

A61   D

Stemetil is a proprietary preparation of prochlorperazine, a phenothiazine used in vertigo and labyrinthine disorders. Stemetil is available as tablets, syrup, injection, effervescent sachets and suppositories. There is no contraindication to the concurrent use of paracetamol and prochlorperazine.

A62   B

Septicaemia occurs when pathogenic micro-organisms or their toxins are present in the bloodstream. Septicaemia is a serious condition characterised by fever, chills, diarrhoea, nausea and vomiting.

A63   C

Hypokalaemia occurs when the plasma-potassium level falls below 3.0 mmol/L. Hypokalaemia may occur following loop or thiazide diuretic therapy. Patients at risk of developing hypokalaemia are often prescribed potassium supplements to counteract the potassium loss caused by the diuretic therapy. Symptoms of hypokalaemia include muscle weakness and cramps. Severe cases may lead to muscle paralysis and respiratory failure.

A64   A

Abdominal pain accompanied by rapid weight loss, vomiting, constipation and unbearable pain warrants referral to exclude peptic ulcers, diverticular disease and carcinoma.

A65 B

Infantile seborrhoeic dermatitis or cradle cap, is a type of eczema common in infants. It presents as scaling and crusting of the scalp within the first three months of life and resolves spontaneously within a year. Management of the condition includes the application and rubbing of almond oil, baby oil, olive oil or clove oil into the scalp, leaving the oil overnight and then washing it off the following day.

A66 A

Lithium is a drug with a narrow therapeutic index and therefore plasma concentrations are regularly monitored. Lithium is used in the prophylaxis and treatment of mania. Concurrent administration of lithium and diuretics, particularly the thiazides, is contraindicated as lithium excretion is reduced, resulting in increased plasma-lithium concentration and hence toxicity.

A67 D

Knee caps, which are indicated for soft tissue support, are not contraindicated in patients taking non-steroidal anti-inflammatory drugs. Knee caps do not result in hypersensitivity reactions.

A68 B

Oilatum bath additive and E45 cream are both emollients which soothe, smooth and hydrate the skin, so are useful in dry skin conditions. Solarcaine gel is a topical anaesthetic preparation containing lidocaine (lignocaine).

A69 B

Cerumol contains chlorobutanol, paradichlorobenzene, and arachis oil. Waxsol contains docusate sodium. Both products are used for ear wax removal. Locorten-Vioform is an ear preparation containing clioquinol (an anti-infective with antibacterial and antifungal properties) and the corticosteroid flumetasone. The preparation is indicated for eczematous inflammation accompanied by otitis externa.

A70   A

Phenergan contains the antihistamine promethazine. Valium contains the benzodiazepine diazepam. Both the antihistamine and the benzodiazepine tend to reduce the blink rate, leading to dry eyes. Logynon is a combined oral contraceptive, which like other oral contraceptives, may cause reduced tolerance because of corneal and eye lid oedema.

A71   C

Pethidine and morphine, used as opioid analgesics, may cause dependence following repeated administration. Zolmitriptan, a 5HT$_1$ agonist used in the treatment of acute migraine attacks, is not associated with dependence.

A72   A

Anti-epileptic drugs, such as phenytoin, carbamazepine and valproate, may lead to neural tube defects if administered during pregnancy. Concurrent administration of folate supplements, such as folic acid, is advised.

A73   E

Vermox is a proprietary preparation of mebendazole, an anthelmintic drug indicated for threadworm or ringworm infections. Mebendazole is administered as a single dose. A second dose can be administered 2–3 weeks after the first dose to prevent re-infection. All members of the family must be treated if the infection is detected in one family member. Use of mebendazole in children under 2 years is not recommended.

A74 C

Patients presenting at the pharmacy complaining of common cold accompanied by pain on coughing and dysphagia warrant referral.

A75 A

Beechams Hot Lemon and Honey is a cold remedy containing paracetamol, ascorbic acid and the sympathomimetic nasal decongestant, phenylephrine. Sympathomimetics mimic the sympathetic system, thereby increasing the heart rate and blood pressure. They may aggravate conditions such as diabetes, hypertension and glaucoma. Patients with hypertension, ischaemic heart disease, hyperthyroidism, diabetes and glaucoma are therefore given topical nasal sympathomimetics rather than systemic sympathomimetics. Both topical and systemic sympathomimetics are contraindicated in patients taking monoamine oxidase inhibitors, because concurrent administration of the two products may lead to a hypertensive crisis.

A76 D

Duphalac is a proprietary preparation of lactulose, an osmotic laxative. Lactulose, which is a semi-synthetic disaccharide, is not absorbed from the gastrointestinal tract and produces an osmotic diarrhoea of low faecal pH, which discourages the proliferation of ammonia-producing organisms.

A77 B

Both phenytoin and theophylline have a narrow therapeutic index.

A78 D

Selective serotonin re-uptake inhibitors such as paroxetine tend to cause less antimuscarinic side-effects and are less toxic in overdose than the tricylic antidepressants, such as amitriptyline. However, selective serotonin re-uptake inhibitors are more likely to cause gastrointestinal disturbances, such as nausea and vomiting, than tricylic antidepressants. Selective serotonin re-uptake inhibitors and tricylic antidepressants are equally effective.

A79   B

The application of a soothing antiseptic cream is the first-choice treatment in patients complaining of severe sunburn. Patients are advised to drink a lot of water to avoid getting dehydrated. A cold shower before going to bed makes the patient feel more comfortable. The application of a local anaesthetic may cause hypersensitivity and is only addressing the pain issue.

A80   A

Dandruff is a form of seborrhoeic dermatitis. Management of dandruff lies with the application of a mild detergent shampoo once or twice a week. Shampoos containing coal tar may be recommended, however, the use of such shampoos is not first-line treatment. Betnovate lotion containing betamethasone, a potent corticosteroid, may be useful in severe dandruff.

A81   B

Calamine lotion is mildly astringent, soothing and has a cooling effect. It is therefore useful in itchy skin conditions, such as chickenpox.

A82   A

Long-term use of oral corticosteroids may result in side-effects, such as peptic ulceration, adrenal suppression and subcapsular cataracts.

A83   C

Sibutramine is a centrally acting appetite suppressant used as an adjunct in the management of obesity. It inhibits the re-uptake of noradrenaline (norepinephrine) and serotonin.

A84   C

Otitis media is inflammation or infection of the middle ear and is not usually associated with back pain. Osteoporosis is a condition occurring mostly in post-menopausal women and is characterised by brittle bones caused by reduced bone mass. It is presented with pain. If it occurs in the vertebral structure the condition may be associated with chronic back pain. Pregnancy may be associated with back pain because of increase in weight and the increased strain.

A85   C

Uniflu contains paracetamol, codeine (opioid analgesic), caffeine (weak stimulant), diphenhydramine (sedating antihistamine) and phenylephrine (nasal decongestant). Patients are advised not to take other paracetamol-containing products, as Uniflu already contains paracetamol. The maximum dose of paracetamol is 4 g (8 tablets) in 24 h.

A86   D

Dequacaine contains the antiseptic dequalinium chloride and the anaesthetic benzocaine. Dequacaine lozenges, indicated for sore throat, cannot be dispensed to diabetic patients as they are not sugar-free.

A87   B

Buscopan is a branded preparation containing hyoscine butylbromide, an antimuscarinic agent that reduces gastrointestinal motility. Antimuscarinic agents are contraindicated in cases of angle-closure glaucoma as they may aggrevate the condition. Hyoscine butylbromide is a quaternary ammonium compound, unlike atropine which is a tertiary ammonium compound. Quaternary ammonium compounds are less lipid-soluble and therefore tend to cause fewer central atropine-like side-effects, whereas peripheral side-effects are more common.

A88 B

Bactroban is the trade name for the topical preparation containing mupirocin. Bactroban is available as nasal ointment or skin ointment. Mupirocin is very effective for treating skin infections caused by Gram-positive organisms but it is not active against Gram-negative micro-organisms. Mupirocin should not be used for longer than 10 days, to avoid development of resistance.

A89 B

Warfarin is an oral anticoagulant. Aspirin may cause gastrointestinal bleeding through its cyclo-oxygenase-1 interference. The concomittant administration of warfarin and aspirin potentiates the risk of bleeding; moreover, internal haemorrhage is very dangerous.

A90 C

Digital thermometers are safer to use in children than glass thermometers as there is no risk of the glass being broken. Digital thermometers tend to be more expensive.

A91 A

Elderly patients must be started on the lowest possible dose of diuretics as they tend to be more susceptible to their side-effects, such as postural hypotension.

A92 D

The extemporaneous mixture of Tinaderm-M and Otosporin ear drops should be discarded after 4 weeks.

A93 A

The combination of Tinaderm-M, an antifungal and Otosporin, a preparation containing antibacterial agents and a corticosteroid, offers a wide spectrum of activity indicated in otitis externa.

A94 E

Diuretics such as bendroflumethiazide (bendrofluazide) tend to cause gout, a condition characterised by a red, swollen great toe caused by the deposition of uric acid at the metatarsophalangeal joint.

A95 D

Gout is a common side-effect of diuretics such as bendroflumethiazide (bendrofluazide).

A96 A

Management of an acute attack of gout involves the use of high doses of non-steroidal anti-inflammatory agents. Colchicine is useful in patients with heart failure where the use of NSAIDs is contraindicated because of water retention. Allopurinol and other uricosuric agents are not indicated for acute attacks as they may aggrevate the condition. The use of an intra-articular corticosteroid injection in gout is unlicensed.

A97 C

Ciprobay is a proprietary preparation of ciprofloxacin, a quinolone.

A98 E

Increasing fluid intake would help flush out urinary tract infections.

A99 A

Ciprofloxacin is a quinolone active against both Gram-positive and Gram-negative organisms. All quinolones must be used with caution in patients taking non-steroidal anti-inflammatory agents as the concurrent administration of the two agents may lead to convulsions. Common side-effects of quinolones include nausea, vomiting and dyspepsia.

A100 C

Urinary tract infections are very commonly caused by Gram-negative bacteria such as *Escherichia coli*, the *Proteus* species and *Pseudomonas* species.

Section 2

Closed-book Questions

Test 4

Questions

Questions 1–38

Directions: Each of the questions or incomplete statements is followed by five suggested answers. Select the best answer in each case.

Q1 Which one of the following is the most appropriate for the management of an upper respiratory tract infection in a patient who is allergic to penicillin?

A ☐ sodium fusidate
B ☐ trimethoprim
C ☐ clarithromycin
D ☐ cefuroxime
E ☐ co-amoxiclav

Q2 The cautionary label 'May cause drowsiness' should be used in all of the following EXCEPT:

A ☐ codeine
B ☐ sumatriptan
C ☐ tramadol
D ☐ co-proxamol
E ☐ diclofenac

Q3   The usual expiration date that should be placed on a cream prepared in a pharmacy is:

A   ☐   1 week
B   ☐   2 weeks
C   ☐   4 weeks
D   ☐   8 weeks
E   ☐   12 weeks

Q4   A 61-year-old retired person receiving 20 mg fluvastatin daily may report:

A   ☐   myalgia
B   ☐   drowsiness
C   ☐   palpitations
D   ☐   constipation
E   ☐   pruritus

Q5   Which of the following is particularly useful in a hypoglycaemic reaction?

A   ☐   sparkling water
B   ☐   still water
C   ☐   sweets
D   ☐   bread
E   ☐   salad

Q6   A pharmacist prepares a saline solution by adding 1 g of sodium chloride in 100 mL water. What is the percentage of sodium chloride present?

A   ☐   10%
B   ☐   1%
C   ☐   0.1%
D   ☐   0.01%
E   ☐   100%

Q7   Thiazide diuretics should usually be avoided in patients with:

A   ☐ hypertension
B   ☐ hypernatraemia
C   ☐ hypercalcaemia
D   ☐ oedema
E   ☐ heart failure

Q8   Alcoholic drink should be avoided with:

A   ☐ amoxicillin
B   ☐ metronidazole
C   ☐ ciprofloxacin
D   ☐ doxycycline
E   ☐ co-trimoxazole

Q9   Which of these components should NOT be included in a preparation during pregnancy?

A   ☐ zinc
B   ☐ iron
C   ☐ folic acid
D   ☐ vitamin A
E   ☐ vitamin E

Q10   A patient is prescribed itraconazole. Which drug may interact with itraconazole?

A   ☐ paracetamol
B   ☐ ibuprofen
C   ☐ digoxin
D   ☐ co-amoxiclav
E   ☐ enalapril

Q11 How many tablets of prednisolone 5 mg should be dispensed to a patient who has been prescribed prednisolone 25 mg for 5 days:

A ☐ 25
B ☐ 125
C ☐ 5
D ☐ 50
E ☐ 45

Q12 All of the following are oral antidiabetic drugs classified as sulphonyl-ureas EXCEPT:

A ☐ glibenclamide
B ☐ chlorpropamide
C ☐ gliclazide
D ☐ tolbutamide
E ☐ metformin

Q13 A proprietary name for ranitidine is:

A ☐ Dyspamet
B ☐ Zantac
C ☐ Tagamet
D ☐ Losec
E ☐ Pariet

Q14 Which preparation could be used systemically in the treatment of acne?

A ☐ azelaic acid
B ☐ clindamycin
C ☐ salicylic acid
D ☐ benzoyl peroxide
E ☐ triclosan

Q15 Which of the following active ingredients is NOT used for the management of cough?

A ☐ codeine
B ☐ dextromethorphan
C ☐ pholcodine
D ☐ vitamin C
E ☐ diphenhydramine

Q16 Tryptizol is classified as a (an):

A ☐ atypical antidepressant
B ☐ tricyclic antidepressant
C ☐ antipsychotic drug
D ☐ antimanic drug
E ☐ hypnotic

Q17 A patient has been prescribed Naprosyn 0.25 g b.d. for 7 days. Naprosyn 500 mg scored tablets are available. How many tablets should be dispensed?

A ☐ 14
B ☐ 12
C ☐ 10
D ☐ 7
E ☐ 4

Q18 The dose of diazepam for children in febrile convulsions is 250 µg/kg. What is the appropriate dose for a child weighing 25 kg?

A ☐ 6250 mg
B ☐ 6.25 mg
C ☐ 62.5 mg
D ☐ 10 mg
E ☐ 625 mg

Q19 Tapeworm infections are caused by:

A ☐ *Taenia solium*
B ☐ tinea pedis
C ☐ *Yersinia pestis*
D ☐ *Candida albicans*
E ☐ *Chlamydia trachomitis*

Q20 Which over-the-counter product is indicated for dyspepsia?

A ☐ Gaviscon
B ☐ Imodium
C ☐ Vermox
D ☐ Buscopan
E ☐ Lomotil

Q21 Which of the following conditions could NOT be caused by a bacterial infection?

A ☐ septicaemia
B ☐ scabies
C ☐ endocarditis
D ☐ peritonitis
E ☐ shigellosis

Q22 Salbutamol:

A ☐ is a selective beta$_2$ adrenoceptor stimulant
B ☐ has a long duration of action
C ☐ should not be used in conjunction with beclometasone (beclomethasone)
D ☐ may cause drowsiness
E ☐ may precipitate oral candidiasis

Q23 Characteristic symptoms of hyperglycaemia include all EXCEPT:

A   ☐ weakness
B   ☐ thirst
C   ☐ visual disturbances
D   ☐ ketonuria
E   ☐ dysuria

Q24 Ergotamine:

A   ☐ may cause tingling of extremities
B   ☐ is used in the prophylaxis of migraine
C   ☐ is included in Migraleve
D   ☐ may be used in hepatic impairment
E   ☐ is a $5HT_1$ agonist

Q25 Drugs used in the treatment of parkinsonism include all EXCEPT:

A   ☐ co-careldopa
B   ☐ amantadine
C   ☐ entacapone
D   ☐ bromocriptine
E   ☐ chlorpromazine

Q26 Oxytocin is used in:

A   ☐ labour induction
B   ☐ premature labour
C   ☐ ductus arteriosus
D   ☐ vaginal atrophy
E   ☐ urinary retention

Q27 Which of the following drugs is NOT liable to cause dry mouth?

A ☐ trihexyphenidyl (benzhexol)
B ☐ cinnarizine
C ☐ imipramine
D ☐ sumatriptan
E ☐ orphenadrine

Q28 Panadol Extra contains paracetamol and:

A ☐ codeine
B ☐ caffeine
C ☐ aspirin
D ☐ ibuprofen
E ☐ diphenhydramine

Q29 Which of the following is of value in the management of furuncles?

A ☐ Hydrocortisyl
B ☐ Fucidin
C ☐ Zovirax
D ☐ Systral
E ☐ Sudocrem

Q30 Which one of the following drugs is NOT likely to cause sensitisation?

A ☐ WaspEze
B ☐ Anthisan
C ☐ BurnEze
D ☐ Solarcaine
E ☐ Hydrocortisyl

Q59 Treatment of gout includes:

1 ☐ indapamide
2 ☐ allopurinol
3 ☐ naproxen

Q60 Gentamicin:

1 ☐ is active against some Gram-positive organisms
2 ☐ is active against anaerobic bacteria
3 ☐ is a cephalosporin

Q61 A patient information leaflet:

1 ☐ is addressed to the prescriber
2 ☐ is only available for medicines presented in bulk dispensing packs
3 ☐ usually includes the recommended International Non-proprietary Name (rINN) of the drug

Q62 Tinnitus:

1 ☐ is the perception of sound in the ears
2 ☐ may be caused by aspirin overdosage
3 ☐ indicates an inflammatory process in the ear

Q63 Common signs of adverse drug reactions include:

1 ☐ urticaria
2 ☐ fever
3 ☐ maculopapular eruptions

Q64 Advantages of selective serotonin re-uptake inhibitors over the tricyclic antidepressants include:

1 ☐ fewer antimuscarinic side-effects
2 ☐ less cardiotoxicity in overdosage
3 ☐ being more effective

Q65 Risk factors for the development of pressure ulcers include:

1 ☐ immobility
2 ☐ incontinence
3 ☐ cough

Q66 Clinical trials:

1 ☐ assess safety and efficacy of a drug in humans
2 ☐ involve different phases
3 ☐ follow good clinical practice standards

Q67 Iron salts:

1 ☐ should be given by mouth unless there are good reasons for using another route
2 ☐ in the form of ferric salts are better absorbed than the ferrous salts
3 ☐ should always be taken on an empty stomach

Q68 Which of the following drug(s) is (are) likely to be prescribed in amenorrhoea?

1 ☐ dydrogesterone
2 ☐ non-steroidal anti-inflammatory drugs
3 ☐ iron supplements

Q69 Disadvantages of depot parenteral preparations include:

1 ☐ increased frequency of dosing compared with oral route
2 ☐ being less effective than other presentations
3 ☐ administration that may not be acceptable to the patient

Q70 Cetirizine:

1 ☐ is a non-sedating antihistamine
2 ☐ is indicated in symptomatic relief of hay fever
3 ☐ is an active metabolite of fexofenadine

Q71 Rubefacients:

1 ☐ act by counter-irritation
2 ☐ should be avoided on broken skin
3 ☐ are exemplified by ketoprofen

Q72 Thyroxine:

1 ☐ is indicated in hyperthyroidism
2 ☐ treatment should not exceed 1 week
3 ☐ should preferably be taken in the morning

Q73 Emollients:

1 ☐ provide a long duration of action
2 ☐ may be applied up to twice daily
3 ☐ are useful in eczema

Q74 Which preparation(s) is (are) available for scalp application?

1 ☐ ketoconazole
2 ☐ coal tar
3 ☐ amoxicillin

Q75   Patients presenting with diarrhoea should be referred if it:

1   ☐ persists for more than 24 h in infants under 1 year
2   ☐ occurs in babies under 3 months
3   ☐ is associated with vomiting

Q76   Preparations that could be recommended to a patient who has athlete's foot include:

1   ☐ salicylic acid
2   ☐ tolnaftate
3   ☐ clotrimazole

Q77   Viral meningitis:

1   ☐ is an infection of brain and spinal cord parenchyma
2   ☐ is not always associated with high fever
3   ☐ is associated with the occurrence of headache

Q78   Which of the following drugs would be effective as a bowel cleanser prior to colonoscopy?

1   ☐ magnesium salts
2   ☐ glycerin
3   ☐ ispaghula husk

Q79   Cough may be associated with:

1   ☐ respiratory infections
2   ☐ lung cancer
3   ☐ smoking

Questions 80–84

Directions: The following questions consist of a first statement followed by a second statement. Decide whether the first statement is true or false. Decide whether the second statement is true or false. Then choose:

A   ☐   if both statements are true and the second statement is a *correct explanation* of the first statement

B   ☐   if both statements are true but the second statement is *NOT a correct explanation* of the first statement

C   ☐   if the first statement is true but the second statement is false

D   ☐   if the first statement is false but the second statement is true

E   ☐   if both statements are false

Directions summarised			
	First statement	**Second statement**	
A	True	True	Second statement is a *correct explanation* of the first
B	True	True	Second statement is *NOT a correct explanation* of the first
C	True	False	
D	False	True	
E	False	False	

 Q80   During pregnancy, diet should consist of foods rich in starch, vitamins and minerals. During pregnancy, food containing sugars, fats and refined carbohydrates should be limited.

Q81 Soft-textured toothbrushes are more efficient in removing plaque than medium-textured brushes. Hard-textured brushes may cause gingival trauma.

Q82 Exercise is contraindicated in controlled angina. Swimming is greatly associated with exercise-induced asthma.

Q83 Support bandages provide support to an injured area during movement. Support bandages reduce risk of infection.

Q84 Calamine lotion may be applied after a jellyfish sting. Jellyfish release histamine that causes erythema.

Questions 85–100

Directions: These questions involve cases. Read the prescription or case and answer the questions.

Questions 85–89: Use the prescription below:

Patient's name ....

Age: 5 years
Panadol 250 mg suppositories
q.d.s.   m. 20
Augmentin 457 mg/5 mL suspension
5 mL b.d.   m. 1 bottle

Doctor's signature ....

Q85 Augmentin is a combination of clavulanic acid and

A ☐ amoxicillin
B ☐ ampicillin
C ☐ co-amoxiclav
D ☐ flucloxacillin
E ☐ pivampicillin

Q86 Augmentin suspension:

1 ☐ should be reconstituted before dispensing
2 ☐ should be agitated before use
3 ☐ should be administered twice daily

A ☐ 1, 2, 3
B ☐ 1, 2 only
C ☐ 2, 3 only
D ☐ 1 only
E ☐ 3 only

Q87 For this patient, dose by rectum of Panadol suppositories is:

A ☐ 125–250 mg up to four times daily
B ☐ 250–500 mg up to four times daily
C ☐ 125–250 mg up to six times daily
D ☐ 60–100 mg up to four times daily
E ☐ up to 4000 mg per day

Q88   Parent may be advised to:

1   ☐ monitor body temperature
2   ☐ keep child well hydrated
3   ☐ discontinue use of Augmentin as soon as symptoms subside

A   ☐ 1, 2, 3
B   ☐ 1, 2 only
C   ☐ 2, 3 only
D   ☐ 1 only
E   ☐ 3 only

Q89   Panadol suppositories may have been preferred to oral suspension because:

1   ☐ there is vomiting
2   ☐ child is reluctant to take medication
3   ☐ there is diarrhoea

A   ☐ 1, 2, 3
B   ☐ 1, 2 only
C   ☐ 2, 3 only
D   ☐ 1 only
E   ☐ 3 only

Questions 90–92: Use the prescription below:

Patient's name   ....
Mobic tablets
1 b.d.   m. 30
Neurorubine-forte
1 b.d.   m. 20
Doctor's signature   ....

NIAID ·

Q90 Mobic could be described as:

1   ☐ antipyretic
2   ☐ anti-inflammatory
3   ☐ analgesic

A   ☐ 1, 2, 3
B   ☐ 1, 2 only
C   ☐ 2, 3 only
D   ☐ 1 only
E   ☐ 3 only

Q91 Neurorubine-forte is prescribed:

1   ☐ as an adjuvant treatment
2   ☐ as a multivitamin preparation
3   ☐ to prevent side-effects of Mobic

A   ☐ 1, 2, 3
B   ☐ 1, 2 only
C   ☐ 2, 3 only
D   ☐ 1 only
E   ☐ 3 only

Q92 The patient could be complaining of:

1   ☐ joint pain
2   ☐ respiratory infection
3   ☐ migraine

A   ☐ 1, 2, 3
B   ☐ 1, 2 only
C   ☐ 2, 3 only
D   ☐ 1 only
E   ☐ 3 only

Questions 93–94: Use the patient profile below:

> *Patient medication file*
>
> **Patient's name** ....
>
> Age   72 years
>
> Medical history   venous thrombosis
>
> Medication record   warfarin 7.5 mg daily
>
> The patient comes to the pharmacy complaining of sore throat, fever and rhinorrhoea.

Q93 What lines of actions would you follow?

1   ☐ dispense paracetamol
2   ☐ dispense a topical nasal decongestant
3   ☐ alter dose of warfarin

A   ☐ 1, 2, 3
B   ☐ 1, 2 only
C   ☐ 2, 3 only
D   ☐ 1 only
E   ☐ 3 only

Q94 What advice should be given?

1   ☐ seek advice from a general practitioner immediately
2   ☐ monitor INR daily
3   ☐ seek advice if condition gets worse

A   ☐ 1, 2, 3
B   ☐ 1, 2 only
C   ☐ 2, 3 only
D   ☐ 1 only
E   ☐ 3 only

Questions 95–100: Use the prescription below:

Patient's name   ....
Spersanicol eye drops
b.d.   m. 1 bottle
Spersanicol eye ointment
nocte   m. 1
Doctor's signature   ....

Q95 Conjunctivitis is inflammation of the:

A   □ eyelid margins

B   □ conjunctiva

C   □ iris

D   □ lacrymal sac

E   □ meibomian glands

Q96 The active ingredient of Spersanicol is:

A   □ gentamicin

B   □ fusidic acid

C   □ oxytetracycline

D   □ dexamethasone

E   □ chloramphenicol

Q97 Common side-effects experienced with Spersanicol may include:

1   □ transient stinging

2   □ agranulocytosis

3   □ photophobia

A   □ 1, 2, 3

B   □ 1, 2 only

C   □ 2, 3 only

D   □ 1 only

E   □ 3 only

Q98 Patient should be advised to:

1 ☐ apply drops morning and midday
2 ☐ apply ointment at night
3 ☐ avoid use of contact lenses

A ☐ 1, 2, 3
B ☐ 1, 2 only
C ☐ 2, 3 only
D ☐ 1 only
E ☐ 3 only

Q99 Eye drops:

1 ☐ are generally instilled into the pocket formed by gently pulling down the lower eyelid
2 ☐ the eye should be kept closed for as long as possible after application
3 ☐ the closure time is preferably 1–2 min

A ☐ 1, 2, 3
B ☐ 1, 2 only
C ☐ 2, 3 only
D ☐ 1 only
E ☐ 3 only

Q100 Spersanicol eye drops:

1 ☐ are sterile before opening
2 ☐ contain a preservative
3 ☐ are available in 30 mL containers

A ☐ 1, 2, 3
B ☐ 1, 2 only
C ☐ 2, 3 only
D ☐ 1 only
E ☐ 3 only

Test 4

Answers

A1   C

First-line treatment in upper respiratory tract infections includes the use of penicillins, cephalosporins and macrolides. Patients who are allergic to penicillins tend to be cross-sensitive to cephalosporins, so are given macrolides such as clarithromycin.

A2   E

The opioid analgesics, such as codeine, tramadol and dextropropoxyphene (found in combination with paracetamol as co-proxamol), may cause drowsiness. Sumatriptan, which is a serotonin agonist, also tends to cause drowsiness. Non-steroidal anti-inflammatory drugs, such as diclofenac, do not cause drowsiness.

A3   C

Extemporaneous preparations, such as creams that are prepared in the pharmacy, have an expiry date of 4 weeks. The creams can be stored at room temperature.

A4   A

Statins, such as fluvastatin, may cause myalgia. Patients are advised to report myalgia immediately.

A5   C

Diabetic patients are advised to carry sweets as a source of sugar in case of a hypoglycaemic reaction.

A6   B

A solution of 1 g of sodium chloride in 100 mL water makes up a 1% w/v solution.

A7   C

Thiazide diuretics act on the beginning of the distal convoluted tubule by inhibiting sodium re-absorption. Thiazide diuretics are indicated in hypertension, and at higher doses to relieve oedema caused by heart failure. Thiazide diuretics lead to hyponatraemia and hypokalaemia. They may cause hypercalcaemia and are therefore avoided in patients with this condition.

A8   B

Concomitant intake of alcohol and metronidazole is potentially dangerous, leading to a disulfiram-like type reaction characterised by intense vasodilation, throbbing headache, tachycardia, sweating and which can lead to death.

A9   D

High concentrations of vitamin A in pregnancy tend to be teratogenic leading to birth defects. Hence vitamin A is contraindicated in pregnancy.

A10   C

Itraconazole is a triazole antifungal, which increases the plasma concentration of digoxin, hence increasing the risk of digoxin toxicity.

A11 A

A patient needs to take five prednisolone 5 mg tablets in a day to make up a daily 25 mg dose. For a five-day supply the patient must be dispensed with 25 prednisolone 5 mg tablets.

A12 E

Metformin is an oral hypoglycaemic agent classified as a biguanide. Metformin decreases gluconeogenesis and increases peripheral utilisation of glucose. Metformin may be used in combination with sulphonylureas. Glibenclamide and chlorpropamide are long-acting sulphonylureas whereas gliclazide and tolbutamide are short-acting and are therefore less likely to be associated with hypoglycaemic attacks.

A13 B

Zantac is a trade name for ranitidine (H_2-receptor antagonist) available as 75 mg, 150 mg and 300 mg tablets. Dyspamet and Tagamet are brands of cimetidine (H_2-receptor antagonist). Losec and Pariet are proprietary preparations of omeprazole and rabeprazole, respectively, both proton pump inhibitors.

A14 B

Topical preparations for the treatment of acne include the use of azelaic acid, salicylic acid, benzoyl peroxide and triclosan. Clindamycin is an antibacterial preparation available for use in the treatment of acne both topically and systemically.

A15 D

Codeine, dextromethorphan and pholcodine are opioid cough suppressants indicated for dry cough. Sedating antihistamines, such as diphenhydramine, tend to have an antitussive action as well. Vitamin C is not used in the management of cough but may be used as a prophylaxis against colds.

A16   B

Tryptizol is a proprietary preparation of amitriptyline, which is a tricyclic antidepressant.

A17   D

The dose 0.25 g is equivalent to 250 mg (half the 500 mg Naprosyn tablet). The patient requires 14 doses of 250 mg Naprosyn tablets and therefore seven 500 mg Naprosyn tablets.

A18   B

The dose for this child is 6250 µg or 6.25 mg (250 µg × 25 kg).

A19   A

Tapeworm infections are caused by *Taenia solium*. Tinea pedis causes the fungal infection known as athlete's foot, *Yersinia pestis* is implicated in plague, *Candida albicans* is responsible for candidiasis while *Chlamydia trachomitis* causes eye infections.

A20   A

Gaviscon is an antacid indicated in dyspepsia. Imodium containing loperamide, and Lomotil containing diphenoxylate and atropine (co-phenotrope) are drugs used in the management of diarrhoea. Vermox contains mebendazole and is indicated in tapeworm infestations, whereas Buscopan contains hyoscine butylbromide, an antispasmodic indicated for the symptomatic relief of gastrointestinal or genitourinary disorders characterised by muscle spasms.

A21 B

Scabies is a skin infection caused by mites. Septicaemia occurs when bacterial micro-organisms or their toxins enter the bloodstream. Endocarditis refers to bacterial infections of the endocardium. Peritonitis occurs when bacterial micro-organisms infect the peritoneum. Shighellosis refers to infections caused by the *Shighella* bacteria.

A22 A

Salbutamol is a selective beta$_2$ receptor agonist indicated in the management of asthma as a bronchodilator relieving acute attacks. It may be used in combination with inhaled corticosteroids such as beclometasone (beclomethasone). Salbutamol acts within a few minutes and tends to be short-acting, unlike salmeterol. Side-effects of salbutamol include tachycardia and palpitations. It does not cause drowsiness and does not precipitate oral candidiasis. Inhaled corticosteroids may precipitate oral candidiasis.

A23 E

Dysuria refers to difficult or painful urination. Dysuria generally indicates urinary tract infections. Symptoms of hyperglycaemia include polyuria (excretion of abnormally large quantity of urine), polydipsia (excessive thirst), visual disturbances, ketonuria and weakness.

A24 A

Ergotamine is an ergot alkaloid indicated for the treatment of migraine. It is contraindicated in hepatic impairment. Side-effects of ergotamine include tingling of extremities, caused by peripheral vasodilation and muscular cramps. Sumatriptan is a serotonin ($5HT_1$) agonist also indicated for the treatment of migraine. Migraleve contains codeine, buclizine and paracetamol.

A25 E

Chlorpromazine is an aliphatic antipsychotic used in schizophrenia and which may exacerbate Parkinson's disease. Co-careldopa is a combination of levodopa and the peripheral dopa-decarboxylase inhibitor, carbidopa. Co-careldopa, amantadine, entacapone and bromocriptine are all indicated in the management of parkinsonism.

A26 A

Oxytocin is administered by slow intravenous infusion for labour induction.

A27 D

Sumatriptan is a serotonin ($5HT_1$) agonist, which does not cause dry mouth. Trihexyphenidyl (benzhexol), cinnarizine, imipramine and orphenadrine all tend to cause antimuscarinic side-effects, including dry mouth, constipation, blurred vision and urinary retention.

A28 B

Panadol Extra contains paracetamol and caffeine, the latter being a weak stimulant.

A29 B

Furuncles (boils) are caused by staphylococci. Fucidin contains fusidic acid which is very effective against boils. Hydrocortisyl contains hydrocortisone, the least potent corticosteroid and which can be applied to the face. Zovirax is a proprietary preparation containing aciclovir (antiviral) indicated for the treatment and prophylaxis of herpes infections. Systral is an antihistamine cream containing chlorphenoxamine. Sudocrem is a barrier preparation containing benzyl alcohol, benzyl benzoate, benzyl cinnamate, lanolin and zinc oxide.

A30   E

Hydrocortisyl (hydrocortisone) is a topical corticosteroid preparation. Corticosteroids are unlikely to cause sensitisation. WaspEze contains benzocaine (local anaesthetic) and mepyramine (antihistamine), BurnEze contains benzocaine, Solarcaine contains lidocaine (lignocaine) (local anaesthetic) and Anthisan is a preparation containing mepyramine (antihistamine). Both antihistamines and local anaesthetics may lead to sensitisation.

A31   D

Otrisal spray contains sodium chloride 0.9% and is effective in relieving rhinorrhoea. Dristan nasal spray and Otrivine nasal drops are proprietary preparations containing the nasal decongestant, oxymetazoline and xylometazoline respectively. Sodium chloride 0.9% may be safer to use in children than topical nasal decongestants as it is less likely to cause side-effects. Locabiotol spray contains fusafungine (antibacterial agent with anti-inflammatory properties) indicated in inflammation and infection of the upper respiratory tract. Bactroban nasal ointment containing mupirocin is indicated for staphylococcal infections.

A32   E

Magnesium hydroxide is a laxative and is not a constituent of oral re-hydration salts, which tend to be recommended for use in diarrhoea, to avoid dehydration. Sodium chloride, glucose, potassium chloride and sodium citrate are required to maintain a proper electrolyte balance and are included in oral rehydration salts.

A33   D

Carbocisteine is classified as a mucolytic as it reduces sputum viscosity and aids its elimination. Carbocisteine is therefore indicated for use in chesty cough. Pholcodine, dextromethorphan and the sedating antihistamines, such as promethazine and chlorphenamine (chlorpheniramine), are indicated in dry cough as cough suppressants.

A34   C

Diclofenac (a non-steroidal anti-inflammatory drug) is marketed as Voltarol oral slow release formulations.

A35   C

Bumetanide is a loop diuretic indicated in oedema. Side-effects of loop diuretics include hypokalaemia, hyponatraemia, hypotension and gout.

A36   C

Baclofen is a skeletal muscle relaxant.

A37   B

Aluminium chloride is a potent antiperspirant indicated for hyperhidrosis, particularly of the feet.

A38 B

Docusate sodium is a preparation used for softening ear wax before removal. Hydrocortisone is a corticosteroid, whereas gentamicin, neomycin and clioquinol are antibacterial agents. Otitis externa may be managed by the use of anti-bacterial preparations used alone or in combination with topical corticosteroids.

A39 B

Symptoms of hepatic failure include accumulation of fluid in the abdomen and lower body leading to ascites, weight loss, muscle wasting, jaundice and anaemia.

A40 C

Peripheral neuropathies is a complication of rheumatoid arthritis.

A41 E

Paget's disease may predispose to secondary osteoarthritis.

A42 C

PMH refers to past medical history.

A43 A

NIDDM refers to non-insulin dependent diabetes mellitus.

A44 E

CAPD refers to continuous ambulatory peritoneal dialysis.

A45   D

Choline salicylate provides analgesic action and is indicated in teething or toothache.

A46   C

Nystatin is a polyene antifungal indicated for the treatment of thrush.

A47   E

Chlorhexidine is an antiseptic mouthwash that inhibits plaque formation on the teeth.

A48   E

Chlorhexidine may cause brown staining of the teeth and therefore patients are advised not to use chlorhexidine on a long-term basis.

A49   E

Fluticasone is a potent corticosteroid which is available as a nasal spray indicated in allergic rhinitis (hay fever) and as an inhaler used in asthma.

A50   A

Prednisolone is a corticosteroid that may be used orally for long-term disease suppression.

A51   C

Hydrocortisone butyrate is marketed as Locoid, a topical corticosteroid available as cream, ointment or lipocream.

A52   D

Prolonged febrile convulsions can be treated by administration of diazepam (benzodiazepine) as a slow intravenous infusion or rectally.

A53   B

Glaucoma is characterised by an increase in intraocular pressure resulting from a decrease in aqueous humour. Clinical features of glaucoma include ocular pain, visual disturbances, headache and sometimes nausea and vomiting.

A54   B

Predisposing factors for low back pain include osteoporosis, trauma and pregnancy.

A55   C

Loperamide is an antimotility drug indicated for diarrhoea. Side-effects of loperamide include skin reactions and abdominal cramps.

A56   B

Sympathomimetics, such as dobutamine and isoprenaline, mimic the sympathetic system. Orphenadrine is an antimuscarinic drug acting as an antagonist to the parasympathetic system.

A57   B

Prophylaxis of angina may be managed by beta-adrenoceptor blockers, such as atenolol, and long-acting nitrates, such as isosorbide dinitrate. Digoxin is a cardiac glycoside that increases the force of myocardial contraction and reduces the conductivity of the heart. Digoxin is indicated as a positive inotrope in heart failure and as an anti-arrhythmic drug in atrial fibrillation.

A58   B

Angiotensin-converting enzyme inhibitors are indicated for use in hypertension and heart failure. Angiotensin-converting enzyme inhibitors have no use in the management of arrhythmias.

A59   E

Treatment of an acute attack of gout is managed by non-steroidal anti-inflammatory drugs, such as naproxen. Drugs such as allopurinol and other uricosurics are not indicated for the treatment of an acute attack of gout as they may prolong the attack. Allopurinol is indicated for prophylaxis of gout and is used on a long-term basis. Indapamide is a thiazide diuretic, which may precipitate an acute attack of gout.

A60   D

Gentamicin is an aminoglycoside active against some Gram-positive bacteria and many Gram-negative bacteria. Gentamicin is inactive against anaerobes. Monitoring of the renal function is important when administering gentamicin.

A61   E

Patient information leaflets are intended to provide information about the medicine to the patient. The leaflets are produced for many medicines whether presented as original packs or patient packs. For medicines presented in bulk dispensing packs, the manufacturer may supply additional copies of the leaflet. Within the European Union, Directive 92/27/EEC outlines the contents of patient information leaflets and the use of the rINN is required.

A62   B

Tinnitus is the perception of sound, such as buzzing, hissing or pulsating noises, in the ears. Tinnitus may be caused by aspirin overdosage, furosemide (frusemide) or gentamicin toxicity. Tinnitus may also be an accompanying symptom of senile deafness, otosclerosis and Meniere's disease.

A63   A

Adverse drug reactions may be characterised by urticaria, fever or maculo-papular rashes.

A64   B

Selective serotonin re-uptake inhibitors (SSRIs) and tricyclic antidepressants are equally effective. However, SSRIs tend to have fewer antimuscarinic side-effects and are less cardiotoxic in case of overdosage. SSRIs tend to cause gastrointestinal side-effects. Both SSRIs and tricylic antidepressants exhibit a time lag before the action of the antidepressants becomes effective.

A65   B

Decreased mobility or immobility and incontinence are risk factors for the development of pressure ulcers. The use of appropriate barrier skin creams may protect against the development of pressure sores, especially in bed-ridden patients.

A66   A

Clinical trials involve different phases of studies of the drug. The aim of clinical trials is to assess safety and efficacy of a drug in humans. Clinical trials must follow good clinical practice guidelines.

A67   D

Iron salts should always be administered by mouth unless there are good reasons for using another route. Ferrous salts are better absorbed than ferric salts. Iron salts may cause gastrointestinal disturbances and are therefore administered after food.

A68   D

Amenorrhoea, which refers to the absence of menstruation, is managed by the administration of progestogen components such as dydrogesterone. Non-steroidal anti-inflammatory drugs are indicated in premenstrual tension. Iron supplements are indicated in menorrhagia (abnormal heavy menstruation).

A69   E

One of the main disadvantages of depot parenteral preparations is that administration of these preparations may not be acceptable to the patient. The depot preparation requires a lower dosing frequency when compared with other dosage forms.

A70   B

Cetirizine is a non-sedating antihistamine drug that may be used for symptomatic relief in allergic rhinitis (hay fever) as it reduces rhinorrhoea and sneezing. Fexofenadine is an active metabolite of terfenadine (another antihistamine).

A71   B

Rubefacients act by counter-irritation produced as a result of local vasodilation, resulting in a warm sensation that masks the pain. Counter-irritants should not be applied on broken skin or before or after taking a hot shower.

Examples of counter-irritants include salicylates, nicotinates, capsicum, menthol and camphor. Ketoprofen is an example of a non-steroidal anti-inflammatory drug that is available as a topical preparation indicated in painful musculoskeletal conditions.

A72 E

Thyroxine (levothyroxine) is indicated in hypothyroidism as a maintenance therapy on a long-term basis. The initial dose must not exceed 100 µg. The usual maintenance dose is 100–200 µg. The dose is decreased in elderly patients. Thyroxine must be taken in the morning.

A73 E

Emollients are useful in eczema as they soothe, smooth and hydrate the skin. The action of emollients tends to be short-lived and therefore they need to be applied frequently.

A74 B

Ketoconazole and coal tar are available as preparations intended for scalp application and are indicated against dandruff.

A75 B

Babies under 3 months with diarrhoea and infants under 1 year presenting with diarrhoea that persists for more than 24 h, require referral. Diarrhoea accompanied by vomiting does not usually warrant referral unless the vomiting is severe.

A76 C

Athlete's foot, tinea pedis, is a condition caused by a fungus. Management of athlete's foot lies within the use of antifungal preparations such as clotrimazole (an imidazole antifungal) and tolnaftate. Salicylic acid is a keratolytic agent indicated for use in treatment of corns, calluses and warts.

A77   C

Viral meningitis refers to inflammation of the meninges. It is characterised by headache, neck stiffness and may be accompanied by fever. Lumbar puncture is required to differentiate between bacterial meningitis and viral meningitis. Viral meningitis, unlike bacterial meningitis, resolves spontaneously and is not life threatening.

A78   D

Magnesium salts are powerful osmotic laxatives, which are useful when rapid evacuation is required and are therefore indicated for bowel cleansing prior to examination of the gastrointestinal tract or before surgery. Glycerine is a stimulant laxative that acts through an irritant action. Ispaghula husk is a bulk-forming laxative, which may be used on a long-term basis but does not bring about a rapid bowel cleansing.

A79   A

Cough may be an accompanying symptom of respiratory tract infections. It is associated with smoking and may be an indication of lung cancer.

A80   B

During pregnancy, a well-balanced diet consisting of starch, fibre, vitamins and minerals is essential. Foods rich in sugar, fats and refined carbohydrates must be limited.

A81   D

Medium-textured brushes are best in removing plaque without causing gingival trauma, as may occur with the hard-texture brushes.

A82   E

Exercise in not contraindicated in controlled angina. However, patients are advised to carry with them glyceryl trinitrate. Swimming is not associated with exercise-induced asthma.

A83   C

Support bandages help brace an injured area during movement but do not reduce risk of infections.

A84   B

Calamine lotion provides a cooling effect that soothes the skin and may be applied after a jellyfish sting. Jellyfish release histamine, which results in erythema and itchiness.

A85   A

Augmentin is a preparation containing the combination known as co-amoxi-clav, that is, amoxicillin (the beta-lactam penicillin) and clavulanic acid, a beta-lactamase inhibitor.

A86   A

Augmentin suspension should be reconstituted with mineral water before dispensing. The parent must be advised to shake the bottle well before use and to administer to the child 5 mL twice daily.

A87   A

The dose of paracetamol suppositories for a 5-year-old child is 125–250 mg four times daily.

A88 B

The parent may be advised to check body temperature, thereby monitoring fever and to keep child well hydrated. Augmentin suspension has to be continued for 7 days.

A89 B

Panadol suppositories may have been preferred either because the patient is reluctant to take the medication or because the patient is vomiting.

A90 A

Mobic is a preparation containing meloxicam, a non-steroidal anti-inflammatory drug. Non-steroidal anti-inflammatory drugs have antipyretic, analgesic, and anti-inflammatory properties.

A91 D

Neurorubine-forte is a vitamin B preparation containing vitamin B_1 (thiamine), vitamin B_6 (pyridoxine) and vitamin B_{12}. It is used as an adjuvant treatment in rheumatoid arthritis.

A92 D

The patient is probably complaining of joint pain and this is the reason why Mobic was prescribed.

A93 B

Paracetamol is indicated as an anti-pyretic and may be safely administered in a patient on warfarin. A topical nasal decongestant is effective for rhinorrhoea (runny nose) and would not interfere with warfarin. Altering the dose of warfarin is only recommended on the basis of results of international normalised ratio (INR) levels.

A94 E

The patient would be advised to seek medical advice if the condition gets worse, as antibacterial agents may be required.

A95 B

Conjunctivitis is inflammation of the conjunctiva. Conjunctivitis may be bacterial, in which case it is accompanied by a purulent discharge, viral or allergic in origin. Generally symptoms include erythema and itchiness.

A96 E

Chloramphenicol, which is a broad-spectrum antibiotic indicated for superficial eye infections, is the active ingredient of Spersanicol products.

A97 D

Spersanicol preparations are only available for topical administration of chloramphenicol. Common side-effects include transient stinging. Agranulocytosis refers to deficiency in neutrophils. Photophobia refers to abnormal intolerance to light.

A98 A

All patients with eye infections are advised to avoid wearing contact lenses. In this case the patient must also be advised to apply the drops in the morning and at midday and to apply the ointment at night.

A99 A

Patients using eye drops are advised to pull down the lower eye lid gently and instil the drops in the pocket formed without touching the dropper with the eyelid. The patient must be advised to keep the eyes closed for as long as possible, closure time being at least 1–2 minutes.

A100 B

All eye drops, including Spersanicol, are sterile before opening and must be discarded within 4 weeks of opening. Spersanicol eye drops contain a preservative and are available in 10 mL containers.

Test 5

Questions

Questions 1–38

Directions: Each of the questions or incomplete statements is followed by five suggested answers. Select the best answer in each case.

Q1 Which one of the following is suitable for the management of lower urinary tract infection in a pregnant woman?

A   ☐   co-trimoxazole

B   ☒   ciprofloxacin

C   ☐   aztreonam

D   ☒   co-amoxiclav

E   ☐   doxycycline

Q2 For which of the following drugs should the label p.c. be used: *— after food.*

A   ☐   salbutamol

B   ☐   tetracycline

C   ☒   prednisolone

D   ☐   dextropropoxyphene

E   ☐   glyceryl trinitrate

Q3 The maximum volume that should be given as a single intramuscular injection at one site is:

A   ☐   20 mL

B   ☐   0.1 mL

C   ☐   1.0 mL

D   ☒   5 mL

E   ☒   2 mL

Q4 A 53-year-old administrative person being treated for hypertension with atenolol 100 mg once daily may report:

A ☐ headache
B ☑ palpitations
C ☐ difficulty with micturition
D ☐ urticaria
E ☒ fatigue

Q5 Non-pharmacological methods that lower blood pressure include:

A ☑ increasing alcohol consumption
B ☐ lowering caffeine intake
C ☒ regular exercise
D ☐ stopping smoking
E ☐ taking small, frequent meals

Q6 A 1% solution of a local anaesthetic contains:

A ☐ 1 mg in 100 mL
B ☑ 1 g in 100 mL
C ☐ 10 mg in 1 mL
D ☐ 1 g in 1 mL
E ☐ 100 mg in 100 mL

Q7 Phenothiazines should usually be avoided in patients with:

A ☐ hypertension
B ☐ anxiety
C ☐ depression
D ☑ closed angle glaucoma
E ☐ insomnia

Q8 Which of the following does not alter a patient's insulin requirements?

A ☐ pregnancy
B ☐ major surgery
C ☒ proton pump inhibitors
D ☐ severe infection
E ☐ food intake patterns

Q9 Which of these drugs cannot be used after delivery to cause the uterus to contract?

A ☒ ritodrine
B ☐ dinoprostone
C ☒ ergometrine
D ☐ oxytocin
E ☐ carboprost

Q10 A patient is being started on amiloride/hydrochlorthiazide tablets. Which drug may interact with the diuretic?

A ☐ salbutamol
B ☒ enalapril
C ☐ diazepam
D ☐ senna
E ☐ atenolol

Q11 Which normal tissue is especially liable to be damaged by cytotoxic drugs?

A ☐ brain
B ☐ cartilage
C ☐ muscle
D ☒ intestinal mucosa
E ☒ bone

Q12 All of the following are antibacterial agents classified as aminoglycosides EXCEPT:

A ☐ gentamicin
B ☐ tobramycin
C ☑ azithromycin
D ☐ amikacin
E ☐ kanamycin

Q13 The proprietary name for bromazepam is:

A ☐ Xanax
B ☒ Lexomil
C ☐ Ativan
D ☑ Valium
E ☐ Mogadon

Q14 Which anti-infective preparation is available only as a topical dosage form?

A ☐ ketoconazole
B ☐ terbinafine
C ☒ mupirocin
D ☑ fusidic acid
E ☐ griseofulvin

Q15 Which of the following is not a nasal decongestant?

A ☐ phenylpropanolamine
B ☒ triprolidine
C ☑ pseudoephedrine
D ☐ phenylephrine
E ☐ oxymetazoline

Q16 Zocor is classified as a (an):

A ☑ statin

B ☐ anthraquinone

C ☐ quinolone

D ☐ salicylate

E ☐ propionic acid derivative

Q17 Calculate the dose of Motilium suspension to be administered to a patient if the paediatric dosing regimen is listed as 2.5 mg/10 kg three times daily. The patient weighs 30 kg. Motilium suspension contains 1 mg of domperidone per mL:

A ☐ 2.5 mL t.d.s.

B ☐ 5 mL t.d.s.

C ☐ 1 mL t.d.s.

D ☐ 75 mL t.d.s.

E ☑ 7.5 mL t.d.s.

Q18 The adult intravenous dose of gentamicin is 2 mg/kg every 8 h. How many milligrams will a 65 kg patient receive daily?

A ☐ 130 mg

B ☐ 1040 mg

C ☑ 390 mg

D ☐ 16 mg

E ☐ 520 mg

Q19 Clotrimazole is indicated to treat infections caused by:

A ☒ Candida albicans

B ☐ Chlamydia trachomatis

C ☐ Neisseria gonorrhoea

D ☑ Staphylcoccus aureus

E ☐ Streptococcus pneumoniae

Q20 Which over-the-counter product is indicated for acute constipation?

A ☐ Imodium
B ☑ Fybogel
C ☐ kaolin and morphine
D ☐ Duphalac
E ☒ Dulcolax

Q21 The rubella virus has the most serious effect on:

A ☐ an elderly patient
B ☑ a pregnant woman
C ☐ a newborn infant
D ☒ a first-trimester fetus
E ☐ an adolescent girl

Q22 Pharmacological effects of calcium-channel blocking agents may include:

A ☐ venoconstriction
B ☒ arteriodilatation
C ☐ hypertension
D ☑ positive inotropic effect
E ☐ increased conduction at the sinoatrial and atrioventricular nodes

Q23 Characteristic symptoms of peptic ulcer disease include all EXCEPT:

A ☒ diffuse abdominal pain
B ☐ pain relief by food
C ☐ pain during the night
D ☑ pain relieved by antacids
E ☐ occasional vomiting

Q24   Metoclopramide

A   ☑ is a dopamine agonist

B   ☐ is not associated with extrapyramidal symptoms

C   ☐ may be used for prophylaxis of travel sickness

D   ☒ adult daily dose is 30 mg

E   ☐ increases oesophageal sphincter contraction

Q25   Drugs used in the treatment of prophylaxis of angina include all EXCEPT:

A   ☐ glyceryl trinitrate

B   ☐ isosorbide dinitrate

C   ☐ nifedipine *ccB* ·

D   ☐ atenolol

E   ☑ losartan *ACE*

Q26   Carbamazepine is used in the treatment of:

A   ☒ trigeminal neuralgia

B   ☐ parkinsonism

C   ☑ hyperthyroidism

D   ☐ hypothyroidism

E   ☐ dementia

Q27   Which of the following drugs is not liable to cause constipation?

A   ☐ codeine

B   ☐ amitriptyline

C   ☐ orphenadrine

D   ☑ senna

E   ☐ tramadol

Q28 Lomotil is a combination of atropine and:

A ☐ diphenhydramine
B ☒ diphenoxylate
C ☐ diphenylpyraline
D ☑ dipyridamole
E ☐ diethyltoluamide

Q29 Which of the following is of value in the management of eczema?

A ☒ Lipobase
B ☐ BurnEze
C ☐ Solarcaine
D ☑ Dovonex
E ☐ Dalacin T

Q30 Which one of the following drugs is likely to cause photosensitivity?

A ☑ amiodarone
B ☐ ferrous sulphate
C ☐ digoxin
D ☐ isosorbide dinitrate
E ☐ propranolol

Q31 A mother comes to the pharmacy with her 3-year-old son who has a cough. Which of the following list of symptoms is most likely to indicate an allergy?

A ☐ nocturnal cough
B ☐ chesty cough
C ☑ rhinorrhoea
D ☐ headache
E ☐ malaise

Q32 Constituents of calamine lotion BP include calamine and:

A ☐ aluminium oxide

B ☑ sodium chloride

C ☒ zinc oxide

D ☐ magnesium hydroxide

E ☐ calcium carbonate

Q33 In gastro-oesophageal reflux disease, which of the following constituents of antacids may be particularly useful:

A ☐ oxetacaine

B ☑ dimeticone

C ☐ chloroform water

D ☐ sucrose

E ☐ lactose

Q34 For which of the following drugs are there significant differences in bioavailability after oral administration:

A ☐ propranolol

B ☑ ampicillin

C ☒ theophylline

D ☐ erythromycin

E ☐ paroxetine

Q35 Common side-effects of itraconazole include all EXCEPT:

A ☐ nausea

B ☑ palpitations

C ☐ dizziness

D ☐ headache

E ☐ abdominal pain

Q36   Dextromethorphan:

A   ☒ is an opioid antitussive
B   ☐ is an analgesic
C   ☑ is a non-opioid antitussive
D   ☐ is available as Silomat syrup
E   ☐ causes diarrhoea as a side-effect

Q37   Topical products for removal of corns and calluses may contain salicylic acid as a (an):

A   ☑ keratolytic agent
B   ☐ bactericidal agent
C   ☐ emollient
D   ☐ local anaesthetic
E   ☐ anhidrotic agent

Q38   Agents that could be recommended for dandruff include all EXCEPT:

A   ☐ selenium sulphide
B   ☐ coal tar
C   ☐ ketoconazole
D   ☑ permethrin
E   ☐ salicylic acid

Questions 39–51

Directions: Each group of questions below consists of five lettered headings followed by a list of numbered questions. For each numbered question select the one heading that is most closely related to it. Each heading may be used once, more than once, or not at all.

Questions 39–41 concern the following conditions:

A ☐ Diabetes
B ☐ Raised intracranial pressure
C ☐ Pregnancy
D ☐ Diverticulitis
E ☐ Oral thrush

Select, from **A** to **E**, which one of the above:

Q39 could be a cause of lower gastrointestinal bleeding D

Q40 could be a cause of early morning headache B

Q41 could be a cause of early morning vomiting C

Questions 42–44 concern the following amino acids:

A ☐ tyrosine
B ☐ serine
C ☐ histidine
D ☐ tryptophan
E ☐ hydroxyproline

Select, from **A** to **E**, the amino acid from which each of the following neurotransmitters is synthesised:

Q42 noradrenaline A ✓

Q43 serotonin B (D)

Q44 histamine C

Questions 45–48 concern the following drugs:

A ☐ folic acid
B ☐ calcium
C ☐ riboflavin
D ☐ magnesium
E ☐ retinol

Select, from A to E, which one of the above:

Q45 is vitamin B_2 _C_ /

Q46 is included in the proprietary product Orovite _B_ x_C_

Q47 is included in the proprietary product Slow-Fe Folic _A_

Q48 is contraindicated during pregnancy _E_

Questions 49–51 concern the following drugs:

A ☐ piperacillin
B ☐ penicillin V
C ☐ penicillin G
D ☐ ampicillin
E ☐ flucloxacillin

Select, from A to E, which one of the above:

Q49 is particularly active against _Pseudomonas aeruginosa_ _A_

Q50 is inactivated by gastric acid _D_ _C_

Q51 is an oral penicillin that is resistant to beta-lactamase _E_

Questions 52–79

Directions: For each of the questions below, ONE or MORE of the responses is (are) correct. Decide which of the responses is (are) correct. Then choose:

A ☐ if 1, 2 and 3 are correct
B ☐ if 1 and 2 only are correct
C ☐ if 2 and 3 only are correct
D ☐ if 1 only is correct
E ☐ if 3 only is correct

Directions summarised				
A	B	C	D	E
1, 2, 3	1, 2 only	2, 3 only	1 only	3 only

Q52   Which of the following is (are) recognised treatments for Crohn's disease?

1 ☐ oral lactulose
2 ☐ oral corticosteroids   *C*
3 ☐ oral sulfasalazine

Q53   Clinical features of hyperthyroidism include:

1 ☐ palpitations
2 ☐ tremor   E x (B)
3 ☐ weight gain

Q54   Predisposing factors for osteoporosis include:

1 ☐ excessive exercise
2 ☐ obesity   C x (E)
3 ☐ advanced age

Q55   Side-effects of application of topical steroids to the skin include:

1   ☐ thickening of the skin
2   ☐ spread of local skin infection   C
3   ☐ striae

Q56   Fibrinolytic agents include:

1   ☐ tranexamic acid
2   ☐ urokinase   C
3   ☐ alteplase

Q57   Drugs useful in the prophylaxis of migraine include:

1   ☐ ergotamine
2   ☐ amitriptyline   E   Ⓒ
3   ☐ propranolol   ×

Q58   Therapeutic uses of benzodiazepines include:

1   ☐ alcohol withdrawal   E
2   ☐ status epilepticus
3   ☐ obsessive compulsive disorder   ×Ⓧ

Q59   Treatment of Parkinson's disease includes:

1   ☐ bromocriptine
2   ☐ orphenadrine   D   ×Ⓑ
3   ☐ moclobemide

Q60   Doxycycline:

1   ☐ is a bacteriostatic   C   ×Ⓡ
2   ☐ is a broad-spectrum antibacterial drug
3   ☐ is effective against chlamydiae

Q61   Which of the following are legal requirements in a prescription?

1   ☐   prescription must be dated
2   ☐   prescriber's signature   B
3   ☐   price of medication

Q62   Tardive dyskinesia:

1   ☐   is particularly prone to occur in the older patient
2   ☐   occurs at a higher frequency with clozapine compared with
         haloperidol   A
3   ☐   is due to reduced dopamine activity

Q63   Causes of acute inflammation include:

1   ☐   bacterial infection
2   ☐   infarction   c
3   ☐   trauma

Q64   Advantages of the combined oral contraceptives over the progestogen-
         only contraceptives are that they are:

1   ☐   suitable for breast-feeding women
2   ☐   less likely to cause deep vein thrombosis
3   ☐   less likely to be associated with irregular vaginal bleeding

Q65   Causes of conjunctivitis include:

1   ☐   viral infection
2   ☐   bacterial infection   C
3   ☐   chlamydiae infection

Q66   Containers used for dispensing medicines should:

1   ☐   always be glass containers
2   ☐   be cleaned with alcohol before use   E
3   ☐   be labelled accordingly

Q67   Clarithromycin:

1   □ cannot be prescribed in conjunction with amoxicillin
2   □ has a shorter half-life than erythromycin
3   □ is used in *Helicobacter pylori* eradication regimens

Q68   Which of the following drugs is likely to be prescribed routinely in the treatment of asthma?

1   □ amoxicillin
2   □ prednisolone
3   □ budesonide

Q69   Disadvantages of inhaled steroids in asthma therapy include:

1   □ hoarseness
2   □ oral candidiasis
3   □ adrenal suppression

Q70   Lactulose:

1   □ acts within 8 h
2   □ acts as an osmotic laxative
3   □ may cause abdominal discomfort

Q71   Hormone replacement therapy:

1   □ provides relief from vasomotor symptoms
2   □ decreases risk of osteoporosis
3   □ increases risk of cardiovascular disease

Q72 Indometacin:

1 ☐ has a superior anti-inflammatory action compared with ibuprofen
2 ☐ rectal administration prevents gastrointestinal tract adverse effects
3 ☐ stimulates cyclo-oxygenase

Q73 Magnesium-containing antacids:

1 ☐ should be used with caution in renal impairment
2 ☐ are exemplified by the proprietary preparation Milk of Magnesia
3 ☐ may cause constipation

Q74 Which preparations are available for administration to the eye?

1 ☐ dexamethasone
2 ☐ betamethasone
3 ☐ docusate sodium

Q75 Accompanying conditions to foot disorders that indicate referral include:

1 ☐ fungal infections
2 ☐ rashes
3 ☐ toenail involvement

Q76 Preparations that could be recommended to a patient who is complaining of sore throat include:

1 ☐ Bradosol lozenges
2 ☐ Corsodyl mouthwash
3 ☐ Otrivine drops

Q77 Amenorrhoea is associated with:

1 ☐ anorexia nervosa
2 ☐ polycystic ovary syndrome
3 ☐ congenital adrenal hyperplasia

Q78 Which of the following drugs would be effective in the treatment of an acute attack of mania?

1 ☐ lithium
2 ☐ haloperidol
3 ☐ flupentixol

Q79 Back pain may be associated with:

1 ☐ osteomalacia
2 ☐ osteoporosis
3 ☐ pregnancy

Questions 80–84

Directions: The following questions consist of a first statement followed by a second statement. Decide whether the first statement is true or false. Decide whether the second statement is true or false. Then choose:

A ☐ if both statements are true and the second statement is a *correct explanation* of the first statement
B ☐ if both statements are true but the second statement *is NOT a correct explanation* of the first statement
C ☐ if the first statement is true but the second statement is false
D ☐ if the first statement is false but the second statement is true
E ☐ if both statements are false

Directions summarised			
	First statement	**Second statement**	
A	True	True	Second statement is a *correct* *explanation* of the first
B	True	True	Second statement is *NOT a correct* *explanation* of the first
C	True	False	
D	False	True	
E	False	False	

Q80 Lorazepam may be used for short-term relief of severe anxiety. Lorazepam is a short-acting benzodiazepine. A ⨉ Ⓑ

Q81 An ultrablock sunscreen preparation always has a sun protection factor of 30. Sunscreen preparations protect the skin from the damage associated with ultraviolet A (UVA). F   E

Q82 A patient with prostatic hypertrophy who has a chesty cough could be advised to use Mucosolvan syrup. Mucosolvan syrup does not contain antihistamine drugs. C   ⨉ Ⓐ

Q83 Eye drops should be discarded after 4 weeks. Eye drops do not contain a preservative. C

Q84 When providing information to the patient, the pharmacist has to convey the information directed to the individual patient's needs. The pharmacist should adjust to the patient's age, personality, and educational background. C ⨉ Ⓑ

Questions 85–100

Directions: These questions involve cases. Read the prescription or case and answer the questions.

Questions 85–89: Use the prescription below:

Patient's name   ....

Age   52 years

Losec 10 mg capsules
o.d.   m. 28
Gaviscon liquid
10 mL q.d.s.   m. 1 bottle

Doctor's signature   ....

Q85   Gaviscon liquid is a combination product containing:

1   ☐ calcium carbonate
2   ☐ alginate
3   ☐ magaldrate

A   ☐ 1, 2, 3
B   ☐ 1, 2 only
C   ☐ 2, 3 only
D   ☐ 1 only
E   ☐ 3 only

Q86   Gaviscon liquid:

1   ☐ should only be used for up to 4 weeks
2   ☐ should be taken after meals
3   ☐ is particularly useful in gastro-oesophageal reflux disease

A   ☐ 1, 2, 3
B   ☐ 1, 2 only
C   ☐ 2, 3 only
D   ☐ 1 only
E   ☐ 3 only

Q87   Losec is a (an):

A   ☐ H$_2$-receptor antagonist, ranitidine

B   ☐ H$_2$-receptor antagonist, cimetidine

C   ☑ proton pump inhibitor, omeprazole

D   ☐ proton pump inhibitor, rabeprazole

E   ☐ prostaglandin analogue, misoprostol

Q88   The patient should be advised to take Losec capsules:

A   ☑ in the morning

B   ☒ once daily

C   ☐ at night

D   ☐ twice daily

E   ☐ as required

Q89   The patient should be advised to:

1   ☐ report occurrence of diarrhoea

2   ☑ reduce weight

C   3   ☑ avoid alcohol intake

A   ☐ 1, 2, 3

B   ☐ 1, 2 only

C   ☐ 2, 3 only

D   ☐ 1 only

E   ☐ 3 only

Questions 90–92: Use the prescription below:

Patient's name   ....

Age   29 years

Fluocinolone acetonide cream
Apply twice daily   m. 1 tube

Doctor's signature   ....

Q90   Which product would you dispense when this prescription is presented?

A   ☑ Synalar
B   ☐ Hydrocortisyl
C   ☐ Travocort
D   ☐ Locoid
E   ☐ Dermovate

Q91   Fluocinolone could be described as:

A   ☑ a mild anti-inflammatory agent
B   ☐ a potent anti-inflammatory agent with anti-infective properties
C   ☒ a potent anti-inflammatory agent
D   ☐ an anti-infective agent
E   ☐ an analgesic agent

Q92   The patient could have:

1   ☐ urticaria
2   ☐ rosacea
3   ☐ dermatitis

A ☐ 1, 2, 3
B ☐ 1, 2 only
C ☐ 2, 3 only
D ☐ 1 only
E ☐ 3 only

Questions 93–95: Use the patient profile below:

Patient medication file

Patient's name   ....

Age   42 years

Allergies   none

Diagnosis   hyperthyroidism

Medication record   Carbimazole 10 mg daily

The patient comes to the pharmacy complaining of sore throat, fever, malaise and dry eyes for the past 2 weeks.

Q93 What line of action would you follow?

1 ☐ dispense Uniflu preparation
2 ☐ dispense hypromellose eye drops
3 ☐ refer patient

A ☐ 1, 2, 3
B ☐ 1, 2 only
C ☐ 2, 3 only
D ☐ 1 only
E ☐ 3 only

After a few days the patient returns with the following prescription:

Patient's name   ....
Cefuroxime tablets 250 mg
b.d.   m. 10
Bronchathiol syrup
10 mL b.d.   m. 1 bottle
Doctor's signature   ....

Q94   Cefuroxime:

1   □ is active against *Haemophilus influenzae*
2   □ is a second-generation cephalosporin
3   □ may cause nausea, vomiting and headache as side-effects

A   □ 1, 2, 3
B   □ 1, 2 only
C   □ 2, 3 only
D   □ 1 only
E   □ 3 only

Q95   Bronchathiol contains a (an):

1   □ antihistamine
2   □ decongenstant
3   □ mucolytic

A   □ 1, 2, 3
B   □ 1, 2 only
C   □ 2, 3 only
D   □ 1 only
E   □ 3 only

Questions 96–100: Use the patient profile below:

Patient medication file

Patient's name ....

Age   26 years

Allergies   penicillin

Diagnosis   tinea corporis

Medication record   Pevaryl PV lotion as directed
                        Lamisil tablets daily

Q96 Tinea corporis is:

A ☐ athlete's foot
B ☐ candidiasis   C
C ☐ ringworm infection
D ☐ thrush
E ☐ dermatitis

Q97 The active ingredient of Pevaryl PV is:

A ☐ clotrimazole
B ☐ ketoconazole   C   x Ⓓ .
C ☐ terbinafine
D ☐ econazole
E ☐ nystatin

Q98 Pevaryl PV lotion was prescribed because:

1 ☐ there is nail involvement   Ⓓ   x Ⓒ .
2 ☐ it will be applied over a large area
3 ☐ it is not occlusive

A ☐ 1, 2, 3
B ☐ 1, 2 only
C ☐ 2, 3 only
D ☐ 1 only
E ☐ 3 only

Q99 Duration of Lamisil treatment in tinea corporis is usually:

A ☐ 12 weeks
B ☐ 2 weeks
C ☐ 4 weeks
D ☐ 6 weeks
E ☐ 1 week

Q100 The pharmacist should advise the patient:

1 ☐ to increase fluid intake
2 ☐ to advise household members about prophylaxis treatment
3 ☐ to continue medications for the entire course of therapy

A ☐ 1, 2, 3
B ☐ 1, 2 only
C ☐ 2, 3 only
D ☐ 1 only
E ☐ 3 only

Test 5

Answers

A1   D

Co-amoxiclav containing the beta-lactam amoxicillin (penicillin) and the beta-lactamase inhibitor clavulanic acid can be safely administered during pregnancy. Co-trimoxazole is contraindicated in pregnancy because of a teratogenic effect. The use of ciprofloxacin (quinolone) in pregnancy is contraindicated because of possible arthropathy in weight-bearing joints of the fetus. Aztreonam (monocyclic beta-lactam antibiotic) is avoided in pregnancy. Doxycyline (tetracycline) is contraindicated because of deposition in bones and teeth of the fetus.

A2   C

Prednisolone tablets must be taken after food to prevent any gastrointestinal irritation and bleeding associated with the systemic administration of steroids.

A3   D

The maximum volume of any substance that can be given as a single intramuscular injection at one site is 5 mL.

A4   E

Common side-effects associated with beta-adrenoceptor blockers, such as atenolol, include fatigue, bradycardia, sleep disturbances, and peripheral vasoconstriction leading to coldness of extremities. Water-soluble beta-blockers, such as atenolol, are less likely to cause sleep disturbances and nightmares than lipid-soluble beta-blockers, such as propranolol.

A5   C

Regular exercise helps in lowering blood pressure especially in obese patients. A sedentary lifestyle is often implicated in cardiovascular disease, such as hypertension. Other non-pharmacological methods that help reduce blood pressure include decrease in sodium intake, moderation of alcohol consumption and avoiding stress.

A6   B

A 1% w/v solution contains 1 g of the active ingredient in 100 mL of the solution.

A7   D

Phenothiazines tend to have antimuscarinic properties and are therefore contraindicated for use in patients with closed angle glaucoma. Antimuscarinics are contraindicated in closed angle glaucoma as they may worsen the condition.

A8   C

A patient's insulin requirements are altered during pregnancy, major surgery, severe infections and altered food intake patterns. Proton pump inhibitors do not affect insulin requirements.

A9   A

Ritodrine relaxes the uterine muscle and is therefore indicated to prevent premature labour. Dinoprostone, ergometrine, oxytocin and carboprost are all indicated to induce or augment labour by inducing uterine contractions and hence can be used to cause the uterus to contract after delivery.

A10 B

Amiloride is a potassium-sparing diuretic, whereas hydrochlorthiazide is a thaizide diuretic that causes loss of potassium. Enalapril is an angiotensin-converting enzyme inhibitor that retains potassium, thereby counteracting the loss of potassium caused by the thiazide diuretic.

A11 D

Cytotoxic drugs are most toxic to rapidly proliferating cells, such as the intestinal mucosa, mucous membranes, skin, hair and bone marrow, leading to nausea and vomiting, stomatitis, alopecia and bone marrow toxicity.

A12 C

Azithromycin is a macrolide having greater activity against Gram-negative organisms than erythromycin but lower activity against Gram-positive organisms. Gentamicin, tobramycin, amikacin and kanamycin are amino-glycosides. Amikacin is a derivative of kanamycin.

A13 B

Bromazepam, a benzodiazepine, is marketed as Lexomil. Xanax is a trade name for alprazolam (benzodiazepine). Ativan is a proprietary name for lorazepam (benzodiazepine); Valium is a proprietary preparation of diazepam (benzodiazepine); Mogadon is a trade name for nitrazepam (benzodiazepine).

A14 C

Mupirocin is an antibiotic agent available only for topical use. It is indicated for use in Gram-positive skin infections. Mupirocin should not be used for more than 10 days, to prevent the emergence of resistance.

A15   B

Triprolidine is an antihistamine. Phenylpropranolamine, pseudoephedrine, phenylephrine and oxymetazoline are nasal decongestants. Nasal decongestants administered systemically are often available in combination with an antihistamine.

A16   A

Zocor is a proprietary preparation containing the statin simvastatin. Statins that competitively inhibit the 3-hydroxy-3-methylglutaryl coenzyme A reductase are more effective in reducing the low-density-lipoprotein cholesterol but less effective in reducing triglyceride concentrations and raising the high-density-lipoprotein cholesterol than the fibrates.

A17   E

The dose for a patient weighing 30 kg would be (2.5 mg × 3) 7.5 mg three times daily. Considering that Motilium suspension contains 1 mg of domperidone per 1 mL, the dose that must be administered is 7.5 mL three times daily.

A18   C

The dose for a patient weighing 65 kg would be (65 kg × 2 mg) 130 mg every 8 h; hence the total daily dose would be 390 mg.

A19   A

Clotrimazole is an imidazole antifungal agent indicated for the treatment of fungal infections caused by *Candida albicans*. The administration of clotrimazole would be of no use in the treatment of infections caused by *Chlamydia trachomatis*, *Neisseria gonorrhoea*, *Staphylcoccus aureus* and *Streptococcus pneumoniae*.

A20   E

Dulcolax is a proprietary preparation of bisacodyl, a stimulant laxative that does not take long to act and is therefore useful in acute constipation. Imodium contains loperamide used in acute diarrhoea. Fybogel contains the bulk-forming laxative ispaghula husk, which takes longer to act but is useful for long-term administration. Kaolin and morphine mixture is indicated in acute diarrhoea. Duphalac contains lactulose, which is an osmotic laxative having a lag time before onset of action.

A21   D

Rubella, also known as German measles, is caused by the rubella virus. Rubella contracted during pregnancy is dangerous to the fetus, especially in the first trimester and may lead to stillbirths, congenital malformations or abortion.

A22   B

Calcium-channel blockers interfere with the inward movement of calcium ions through the cell membrane channels. This results in reduction of myocardial contractility (hence negative inotropes), reduction of cardiac output and arteriolar vasodilatation. The dihydropyridine group, such as nifedipine and amlodipine, which may be used in the management of hypertension, are very effective as arterial vasodilators, whereas diltiazem and verapamil are very effective in reducing atrioventricular conduction.

A23   A

Localised upper abdominal pain is the most common symptom of peptic ulcer disease. The pain is relieved by antacids, proton pump inhibitors and H_2 antagonists. The pain may or may not be relieved by food and is often worse during the night. Peptic ulceration may be accompanied by occasional vomiting, anorexia and weight loss. Diffuse abdominal pain is not a characteristic symptom of peptic ulcer disease.

A24   D

Metoclopramide is a dopamine antagonist indicated as an anti-emetic in vomiting associated with gastrointestinal, hepatic and biliary disorders and in vomiting associated with cytotoxics and radiotherapy. Metoclopramide, which enhances gastric emptying, is not effective in motion sickness. The adult dose of metoclopramide is 10 mg three times daily. Metoclopramide, being a dopamine antagonist, may result in extrapyramidal symptoms, particularly in young adults.

A25   E

Losartan is an angiotensin II receptor antagonist indicated as an alternative to angiotensin-converting enzyme inhibitor drugs in the management of hypertension. Treatment and prophylaxis of angina is managed by nitrates, such as glyceryl trinitrate and isosorbide dinitrate; and by beta-adrenoceptor blockers, such as atenolol and by calcium-channel blockers, such as long-acting nifedipine.

A26   A

Carbamazepine is an anti-epileptic, which may also be used in the treatment of trigeminal neuralgia. Monitoring of carbamazepine plasma concentrations is required if high doses are administered as carbamazepine tends to be an autoinducer, meaning that the half-life is shortened following repeated administration of the drug.

A27   D

One of the main side-effects of opioid analgesics, such as codeine and tramadol, is constipation. Amitriptyline (tricyclic anti-depressant) and orphenadrine tend to have antimuscarinic properties, resulting in side-effects such as constipation. Senna is a stimulant laxative indicated in constipation.

A28 B

Lomotil is an antidiarrhoeal product containing the combination known as co-phenotrope, consisting of atropine and diphenoxylate. Diphenoxylate is an opioid and similar to morphine and loperamide; it increases the tone of the gastrointestinal muscle and reduces the motility within the gastrointestinal tract leading to constipation. To avoid possible development of dependence on diphenoxylate, it is combined with atropine, the antimuscarinic side-effects of which deter patients from abusing diphenoxylate.

A29 A

Eczema is managed by emollients and topical corticosteroids. Lipobase is an emollient preparation and is therefore indicated in eczema. BurnEze is a product containing the local anaesthetic benzocaine, and Solarcaine gel is a product containing lidocaine (lignocaine). Dovonex contains calcipotriol, used in psoriasis. Dalacin T contains clindamycin, used in acne.

A30 A

Amiodarone is an anti-arrhythmic drug indicated in supraventricular and ventricular arrhythmias. One of the main side-effects is photosensitivity and patients are advised to avoid exposure to sunlight and use sun protection factors.

A31 C

Rhinorrhoea and sneezing are characteristic symptoms of allergic rhinitis (hay fever). Nocturnal cough in children is indicative of asthma. Chesty cough indicates a bacterial upper respiratory tract infection. Headache and malaise are accompanying symptoms of common colds. Headache may also develop in allergic rhinitis, because of congested sinuses.

A32 C

Calamine lotion is a combination of calamine and zinc oxide. It is mildly astringent and imparts a soothing antipruritic effect. Calamine lotion is cheap and effective with few restrictions on its use.

A33 B

Activated dimeticone (simethicone) acts as an antifoaming agent thereby reducing flatulence and being effective in gastro-oesophageal reflux disease. Oxetacaine is a local anaesthetic, which is added to antacids to improve symptom relief. Chloroform water is a traditional preparation to reduce colic. Sucrose and lactose are sugars with no effect on gastro-oesophageal reflux disease.

A34 C

Theophylline is a narrow therapeutic index drug with significant difference in bioavailability following oral administration. The half-life of the drug is increased by heart failure, cirrhosis and viral infections, in elderly patients, and by certain drugs, such as cimetidine, ciprofloxacin, oral contraceptives and fluvoxamine. The half-life is decreased in smokers, chronic alcoholism, and by certain drugs, such as phenytoin, rifampicin and carbamazepine.

A35 B

Itraconazole is a triazole antifungal causing side-effects, such as nausea, abdominal pain, dizziness and headache. Itraconazole does not lead to palpitations; however, it may lead to heart failure and hence itraconazole is administered with caution to patients at risk of heart failure.

A36 A

Dextromethorphan is an opioid antitussive similar in action to codeine and pholcodine. Codeine and pholcodine are considered to be more potent than dextromethorphan. Dextromethorphan tends to cause less constipation and dependence than codeine. Silomat syrup contains clobutinol.

A37   A

Topical products for removal of corns and calluses often contain salicylic acid at a concentration of between 11% and 50% as a keratolytic agent in combination with lactic acid, the latter intended to aid absorption.

A38   D

Selenium sulphide, coal tar, ketoconazole and salicylic acid are agents that can be used in dandruff. Permethrin is an insecticide indicated in the eradication of head lice. Permethrin is available as alcoholic or aqueous lotions.

A39   D

Diverticulitis refers to the extension of mucosal pouches outwards from the external muscle wall into the gastrointestinal tract. Diverticulitis is accompanied by colicky pain lasting for a few days. The condition is accompanied by constipation or diarrhoea and blood in stools.

A40   B

Raised intracranial pressure could be a cause of early morning headache. Early morning headache could also be triggered by sinusitis, tension or muscle spasm.

A41   C

Pregnancy is a common cause of early morning vomiting. The condition is referred to as morning sickness and may be relieved by taking dry biscuits on waking up.

A42   A

Tyrosine is the amino acid precursor of the sympathetic neurotransmitter noradrenaline.

A43   D

Tryptophan is the amino acid precursor of the neurotransmitter serotonin.

A44   C

Histidine is the amino acid precursor of the neurotransmitter histamine.

A45   C

Vitamin B_2 is another name for riboflavin.

A46   C

Orovite is a proprietary preparation containing vitamin B_1 (thiamine), vitamin B_2 (riboflavin), vitamin B_6 (pyridoxine), nicotinamide and ascorbic acid.

A47   A

Slow-Fe Folic is a proprietary preparation containing iron and folic acid. It is indicated in pregnant women who are at risk of developing iron and folic acid deficiency.

A48   E

Retinol is contraindicated for use in pregnancy because of its teratogenic effect.

A49   A

Piperacillin is classified as a ureidopenicillin. It is active against *Pseudomonas aeruginosa*.

A50   C

Penicillin G, also referred to as benzylpenicillin, is inactivated by gastric acid and is therefore available only for injection.

A51   E

Flucloxacillin is an oral beta-lactam penicillin, which is resistant to the enzyme beta-lactamase and is therefore indicated in infections caused by penicillin-resistant organisms.

A52   C

Treatment of Crohn's disease is based on the administration of oral cortico-steroids, to attain remission. Oral aminosalicylates, such as oral sulfasalazine, are indicated for long-term use as maintenance treatment. Oral corticosteroids are not indicated for maintenance treatment because of their side-effects.

A53   B

Patients with hyperthyroidism tend to have enhanced metabolism leading to weight loss, tremor and palpitations. Propranolol may be indicated to reduce the sympathetic symptoms, such as tremor and palpitations.

A54   E

Advanced age is a common predisposing factor to the development of osteo-porosis.

A55   C

Topical application of corticosteroids may lead to spreading of local skin infections, striae and thinning of the skin. Topical preparations containing corticosteroids should not be applied for more than 7 days.

A56   C

Fibrinolytic agents, such as alteplase and urokinase, activate plasminogen to plasmin, which in turn degrades fibrin thereby breaking the thrombus and acting as thrombolytics. Fibrinolytic agents are indicated in acute myocardial infarction, venous thrombosis and embolism. Tranexamic acid is an anti-fibrinolytic agent consequently inhibiting fibrinolysis and bleeding.

A57   C

Ergotamine is an ergot derivative indicated for the treatment of migraine. Amitriptyline and propranolol can be used for the prophylaxis of migraine.

A58   A

All benzodiazepines are indicated in obsessive compulsive disorders. Diazepam and lorazepam are effective in status epilepticus, whereas chlordiazepoxide is indicated in alcohol withdrawal.

A59   B

Bromocriptine is a dopamine agonist acting by direct stimulation of the dopamine receptors. In Parkinson's disease, it is reserved for use in patients who are intolerant to levodopa or in whom levodopa alone is not sufficient. Orphenadrine is an antimuscarinic indicated in Parkinson's disease. Antimuscarinics tend to be more effective than levodopa in targeting tremor rather than rigidity and bradykinesia. Moclobemide is an antidepressant referred to as a reversible monoamine oxidase inhibitor (RIMA) type A.

A60   A

Doxycyline is a tetracycline antibiotic. All tetracylines are bacteriostatic, have a broad spectrum and are the treatment of choice for infections caused by *Chlamydia* and *Rickettsia* and in brucellosis. Doxycyline and minocyline are the only two tetracyclines that may be administered in renal impairment.

A61   B

Prescribers are expected to include the date of issue of the prescription and their signature.

A62   D

Tardive dyskinesia refers to uncontrollable facial movements. It is more likely to occur in the elderly. Tardive dyskinesia is commonly associated with the use of antipsychotic drugs, such as haloperidol. The atypical antipsychotics, such as clozapine, olanzapine, risperidone and quetiapine are less likely to cause tardive dyskinesia.

A63   A

Acute inflammation may be due to bacterial infection, infarction and trauma.

A64   E

Combined oral contraceptives are less likely to be associated with irregular vaginal bleeding than progestogen-only contraceptives. However, they are less suitable for smokers and breast-feeding women. They are more likely to cause deep-vein thrombosis than progestogen-only contraceptives.

A65   A

Conjunctivitis may be caused by viral infections, bacterial infections or infections caused by *Chlamydia*. Conjunctivitis caused by bacterial infections tends to be accompanied by a coloured discharge.

A66   E

Containers used for dispensing should always be labelled accordingly, preferably also with cautionary labels. Child-resistant containers may be difficult to use by elderly patients. Not all containers should be cleaned with alcohol before use as the medicine may interact with the alcohol.

A67   E

Clarithromycin is a macrolide that has a longer half-life than erythromycin so is administered twice daily. Clarithromycin is more active against Gram-positive organisms than erythromycin. Clarithromycin may be used in combination with amoxicillin, for example, as part of triple therapy used for the eradication of *Helicobacter pylori*.

A68   E

Asthma is managed by the use of an inhaled bronchodilator prescribed on an as-required (p.r.n.) basis to relieve acute attacks and administration of an inhaled corticosteroid as maintenance therapy. Budesonide is available as inhaled corticosteroid. Oral prednisolone is indicated in the treatment of severe, uncontrolled asthma for short-term periods.

A69 B

Side-effects and disadvantages of inhaled corticosteroids include hoarseness and oral candidiasis. Patients on inhaled corticosteroids are advised to rinse their mouth with water after using the inhaler, to reduce the occurrence of such side-effects. Adrenal suppression is a side-effect more likely to be associated with the long-term use of oral corticosteroids.

A70 C

Lactulose is an osmotic laxative acting by retaining fluid in the bowel. It takes a long time to act, generally up to 48 h, and may cause abdominal discomfort.

A71 B

Hormone replacement therapy provides relief from vasomotor symptoms, decreases the risk of oesteoporosis and decreases the risk of cardiovascular disease in post-menopausal women.

A72 D

Indometacin, which is a non-steroidal anti-inflammatory drug, inhibits the enzyme cyclo-oxygenase implicated in inflammatory reactions. Indometacin is superior in action to ibuprofen and tends to have a higher side-effect profile, including headache, diarrhoea and gastrointestinal disturbances. Rectal administration reduces but does not prevent gastrointestinal tract disturbances.

A73 B

Magnesium-containing antacids, such as Milk of Magnesia, must be used with caution in renal impairment as the absorption of magnesium may lead to hypermagnesaemia with serious cardiovascular and neurological consequences. Magnesium-containing antacids tend to have a laxative effect and are often marketed in combination with aluminium-containing antacids to counteract the constipating effect of the aluminium antacid.

A74   B

Dexamethasone and betamethasone are corticosteroids available for topical application in eye products. Docusate sodium is indicated for ear wax removal.

A75   E

Referral for foot conditions is indicated in toenail involvement, diabetic patients and where foot colour and appearance are abnormal.

A76   D

Bradosol lozenges contain the antiseptic benzalkonium. Preparations for sore throat contain antiseptics or anaesthetic or a combination of the two. Corsodyl mouthwash contains chlorhexidine, which is effective in periodontal disease. However, frequent use of Corsodyl should be discouraged as chlorhexidine stains the teeth. Otrivine drops are a topical nasal decongestant preparation containing xylometazoline, indicated in rhinorrhoea.

A77   A

Amenorrhoea, which refers to the absence of menstruation, is associated with anorexia nervosa, polycystic ovary syndrome and congenital adrenal hyperplasia. The condition requires referral.

A78   C

Antipsychotic drugs, such as flupentixol and haloperidol are the mainstay of treatment for acute attacks of mania. Lithium is not indicated as it may take a few days before the drug exerts an effect. Lithium may be given concomitantly with an antipsychotic drug.

A79 C

Back pain may be associated with osteoporosis and pregnancy. Osteomalacia refers to insufficient mineralisation of the bones, resulting in soft bones.

A80 B

Lorazepam is a short-acting benzodiazepine. Both short-acting and long-acting benzodiazepines, such as diazepam, may be indicated for short-term relief of severe anxiety.

A81 E

Sunscreen preparations tend to contain substances that protect the skin against sunburn caused by ultraviolet B (UVB) rays. UVA rays are associated with long-term skin damage. Sunscreen preparations contain a variety of sun protection factors but not necessarily a factor of 30.

A82 A

Mucosolvan syrup contains ambroxol, a mucolytic agent used in chesty cough. Antihistamines tend to have antimuscarinic properties, resulting in urinary retention and are therefore contraindicated in prostatic hypertrophy.

A83 C

Eye drops should be discarded 4 weeks after opening because of loss of sterility of the product. Eye drops do contain preservatives.

A84 B

It is important to convey information about medications as directed according to the needs of each patient. Moreover the pharmacist must use appropriate, simple language and adjust according to the patient's age, personality and educational background.

A85 B

Gaviscon liquid is an antacid preparation containing calcium carbonate, alginate and sodium bicarbonate.

A86 C

Gaviscon liquid should be administered four times daily after food. It is particularly useful in gastro-oesophageal reflux disease due to the alginate component which tends to act as an antifoaming agent relieving flatulence.

A87 C

Losec is a trade name for omeprazole, a proton pump inhibitor which inhibits gastric acid secretion by blocking the proton pump.

A88 B

According to the prescription, the patient should be advised to take one Losec capsule daily.

A89 C

The patient probably has gastro-oesophageal reflux. Weight reduction and avoidance of alcohol help to reduce the occurrence of gastro-oesophageal reflux.

A90 A

Synalar is a topical proprietary preparation containing fluocinolone acetonide, a corticosteroid.

A91 C

Fluocinolone is a potent corticosteroid anti-inflammatory agent.

A92 E

Dermatitis is a common inflammatory condition, which may require the use of a potent topical corticosteroid. Rosacea is a skin disorder whereby the blood vessels of the face enlarge giving the face a flushed appearance. Urticaria refers to the appearance of red wheals which may be due to an allergy.

A93 C

Carbimazole tends to cause neutropenia and patients are advised to report any sore throat to the pharmacist for referral. Blood counts would be required. Dry eyes are a consequence of hyperthyroidism and hypromellose eye drops could be recommended for the relief of dry eyes.

A94 A

Cefuroxime is a second-generation cephalosporin with enhanced activity against *Haemophilus influenzae*, a Gram-negative organism. Side-effects include nausea, vomiting and headache.

A95 E

Bronchathiol syrup contains carbocisteine, a mucolytic agent.

A96 C

Tinea corporis is ringworm infection.

A97 D

The active ingredient of Pevaryl PV is the imidazole antifungal, econazole.

A98 C

An antifungal in the form of lotion was prescribed because a large area is involved and lotion is easy to apply and is not occlusive.

A99 C

Treatment for tinea corporis takes about 4 weeks and adherence to the treatment is important for an effective outcome.

A100 E

The pharmacist should strongly advise the patient to continue with the prescribed medications for the entire course so that treatment is effective. Measures to avoid contamination of household members could be followed but prophylaxis treatment is not usually recommended.

Test 6

Questions

Questions 1–37

Directions: Each of the questions or incomplete statements is followed by five suggested answers. Select the best answer in each case.

Q1 Which one of the following components of cough preparations is NOT an antitussive?

- A ☑ diphenhydramine *– antihistamine*
- B ☐ dextromethorphan
- C ☐ pholcodine
- D ☒ ammonium chloride
- E ☐ codeine phosphate

Q2 When advising a patient on the correct use of eye drops, which one of the following statements is *incorrect*?

- A ☐ tilt your head back and pull down the lower lid of your eye with the index finger
- B ☐ hold the tip of the dropper against the lower lid
- C ☐ gently squeeze the dropper so that the correct number of drops are released
- D ☐ close the eye for two to three minutes and wipe any excess liquid from your face with a tissue
- E ☐ replace and tighten cap

Q3   Topical products for acne may contain benzoyl peroxide as a (an):

A ☑ antimicrobial
B ☐ emollient
C ☒ keratolytic
D ☐ bactericidal
E ☐ retinoid

Q4   Naproxen is classified as:

A ☐ a sulphonamide
B ☐ a corticosteroid
C ☑ a propionic acid derivative
D ☐ an anthraquinone
E ☐ an econazole

Q5   5000 mg equals 0.005:

A ☐ grams
B ☑ kilograms
C ☐ micrograms
D ☐ centigrams
E ☐ nanograms

Q6   Calculate the dose of a drug to be administered to a patient if the dosing regimen is listed as 5 mg/kg per day in divided doses every 8 h. The patient weighs 67 kg:

A ☐ 67 mg t.d.s.
B ☐ 42 mg t.d.s.
C ☑ 335 mg t.d.s.
D ☐ 14 mg t.d.s.
E ☒ 112 mg t.d.s.

Q7 A pharmacist is required to dispense 30 g of 0.5% hydrocortisone ointment. The pharmacist has available a hydrocortisone ointment 1%. How
many grams of the 1% ointment could be diluted with white soft paraffin
to prepare this order?

A ☑ 15 g $\frac{30 \times 0.5}{1} = 15.$
B ☐ 30 g
✓ C ☐ 0.15 g
D ☐ 0.5 g
E ☐ 1.5 g

Q8 Which one of the following agents is indicated for use as an anti-emetic
agent?

A ☐ docusate sodium
B ☐ lansoprazole
C ☑ ondansetron
D ☐ ranitidine
E ☐ mebeverine

Q9 The product which may be recommended safely for use by an infant
with nasal congestion is:

A ☐ topical pseudoephedrine
B ☑ normal saline
C ☐ systemic pseudoephedrine
D ☐ cetirizine
E ☐ mefenamic acid

Q10 A major target organ for gentamicin toxicity is the:

A ☐ heart
B ☑ liver
C ☒ kidney
D ☐ stomach
E ☐ brain

Q11   Common side-effects of salbutamol include all EXCEPT:

A   ☐ fine tremor
B   ☐ tachycardia
C   ☐ headache
D   ☑ constipation
E   ☐ muscle cramps

Q12   Bezafibrate is a (an):

A   ☑ lipid-regulating drug
B   ☐ antihypertensive
C   ☐ laxative
D   ☐ antispasmodic
E   ☐ calcium-channel blocker

Q13   What is the maximum adult daily dose for Otrivine drops?

A   ☒ three drops into each nostril four times daily
B   ☑ one drop into each nostril three times daily
C   ☐ three drops into each nostril six times daily
D   ☐ one drop into each nostril twice daily
E   ☐ six drops into each nostril three times daily

Q14   Citalopram is a (an):

A   ☑ SSRI
B   ☐ TCA
C   ☐ antipsychotic
D   ☐ benzodiazepine
E   ☐ MAOI

Q15 An electrolyte supplement used to replenish electrolytes lost as a consequence of diarrhoea is:

A ☐ Picolax

B ☐ Ensure

C ☒ Dioralyte

D ☐ Citramag

E ☐ Kay-Cee-L

Q16 An example of a topical preparation containing an antibacterial agent in combination with a corticosteroid is:

A ☐ Eurax

B ☒ Fucicort

C ☐ Dermovate

D ☒ Nerisone

E ☐ Pevaryl

Q17 What is the recommended dose of paracetamol for a child aged 5 years?

A ☒ 250 mg every 4–6 h

B ☒ 125 mg every 4–6 h

C ☐ 500 mg every 4–6 h

D ☐ 250 mg every 6–8 h

E ☐ 125 mg every 6–8 h

Q18 Levonorgestrel is a (an):

A ☒ progestogen

B ☐ oestrogen

C ☐ prostaglandin

D ☐ gonadorelin analogue

E ☐ glucocorticoid

Q19 Aciclovir is indicated for the treatment of:

A ☑ cold sores

B ☐ erythema

C ☐ measles

D ☐ rubella

E ☐ pruritus

Q20 Carbimazole is used in the treatment of:

A ☐ diabetes mellitus

B ☑ hyperthyroidism

C ☐ hypothyroidism

D ☐ carcinoma

E ☐ ulcerative colitis

Q21 Which one of the following antihistamines is least likely to cause sedation?

A ☐ diphenhydramine

B ☒ desloratadine

C ☐ chlorphenamine (chlorpheniramine)

D ☐ promethazine

E ☑ alimemazine (trimeprazine)

Q22 Alginic acid is found in some antacid preparations. The primary function is to:

A ☐ act as an antifoaming agent

B ☑ accelerate gastric emptying

C ☒ prevent refluxing into the oesophagus

D ☐ act as an antimuscarinic

E ☐ act as a flavouring agent

Q23 The use of a suspension as a parenteral preparation is contraindicated when the route of administration is:

A ☐ subcutaneous
B ☐ intramuscular
C ☑ intravenous
D ☐ intradermal
E ☐ intra-articular

Q24 Preparations used for infant colic contain:

A ☑ activated dimeticone
B ☐ metoclopramide
C ☐ domperidone
D ☐ cisapride
E ☐ ranitidine

Q25 Which of the following antibacterial drugs is NOT available for oral administration?

A ☐ tetracycline
B ☑ fusidic acid
C ☒ gentamicin
D ☐ erythromycin
E ☐ ciprofloxacin

Q26 All of the following are viral infections EXCEPT:

A ☐ chickenpox
B ☑ tinea pedis
C ☐ hepatitis
D ☐ mumps
E ☐ rubella

Q27   A tourist comes to the pharmacy asking for a sun lotion for sun protection. Which product would you recommend?

A   ☐ tanning oil SPF 4
B   ☐ tanning oil SPF 8
C   ☐ lotion SPF 2
D   ☐ lotion SPF 6
E   ☑ lotion SPF 8

Q28   Bioavailability describes the relative amount of drug that reaches the:

A   ☐ kidney
B   ☑ systemic circulation
C   ☐ liver
D   ☐ stomach
E   ☐ small intestine

Q29   When a drug is administered as a solid oral dosage form, the first process which occurs is:

A   ☐ absorption
B   ☑ disintegration
C   ☐ dissolution
D   ☐ ionisation
E   ☐ metabolism

Q30   Which of the following agents is NOT employed in the treatment of depression?

A   ☑ lorazepam
B   ☐ imipramine
C   ☐ paroxetine
D   ☐ venlafaxine
E   ☐ moclobemide

Q31 For which of the following is immunisation NOT provided to children:

A   ☐ measles

B   ☐ mumps

C   ☑ infectious mononucleosis

D   ☐ rubella

E   ☐ diphtheria

Q32 Rubella virus has the most serious effect on:

A   ☑ a pregnant woman

B   ☐ an adolescent girl

C   ☒ a fetus

D   ☐ a diabetic patient

E   ☐ a newborn infant

Q33 The first line of treatment of rheumathoid arthritis is:

A   ☐ sodium aurothiomalate

B   ☐ paracetamol

C   ☑ indometacin – NSAID .

D   ☒ diclofenac

E   ☐ dexamethasone

Q34 Which of the following drugs should be used with utmost caution in a patient who had a severe allergic reaction to penicillin?

A   ☐ clindamycin

B   ☐ ketoconazole

C   ☑ cefaclor

D   ☐ vancomycin

E   ☐ erythromycin

Q35 Which of the following non-steroidal anti-inflammatory drugs would be of particular use in a patient with arthritis who also complains of dyspepsia from time to time?

A ☐ diclofenac potassium

B ☐ aspirin

C ☐ indometacin

D ☑ meloxicam

E ☐ diclofenac sodium

Q36 Paracetamol overdose is most likely to cause:

A ☐ renal damage

B ☐ tinnitus

C ☑ hepatic necrosis

D ☐ seizures

E ☐ ataxia

Q37 The drug of choice in prolonged febrile convulsions is:

A ☐ carbamazepine

B ☑ diazepam

C ☐ phenytoin

D ☐ paracetamol

E ☐ mefenamic acid

Questions 38–61

Directions: Each group of questions below consists of five lettered headings followed by a list of numbered questions. For each numbered question select the one heading that is most closely related to it. Each heading may be used once, more than once, or not at all.

Questions 38–40 concern the following corticosteroids:

A ☐ hydrocortisone
B ☐ hydrocortisone butyrate
C ☐ fluocinolone
D ☐ fluticasone
E ☐ clobetasone

Select, from A to E, which one of the above:

Q38 is available orally D x(A)

Q39 is the least potent A

Q40 is available for inhalation D

Questions 41–43 concern the following diuretics:

A ☐ furosemide (frusemide)
B ☐ bendroflumethiazide (bendrofluazide)
C ☐ spironolactone
D ☐ polythiazide
E ☐ indapamide

Select, from A to E, which one of the above:

Q41 inhibits re-absorption from ascending loop of Henle in renal tubule A

Q42 should be used with caution in patients with enlarged prostate A

Q43 is a potassium-sparing diuretic C

Questions 44–47 concern the following antipsychotic drugs:

A ☐ chlorpromazine
B ☐ flupentixol
C ☐ haloperidol
D ☐ thioridazine
E ☐ prochlorperazine

Select, from A to E, which one of the above:

Q44 is associated with pronounced sedative effects E x Ⓐ

Q45 is characteristically associated with a low incidence of extrapyramidal side-effects B · x Ⓓ

Q46 is classified as a thioxanthene antipsychotic drug D x Ⓑ

Q47 is exemplified by the proprietary product Largactil A

Questions 48–50: Match the lettered generic name most closely corresponding to the numbered proprietary (brand) name:

A ☐ senna
B ☐ ispaghula husk
C ☐ loperamide
D ☐ sodium picosulfate
E ☐ bisacodyl

Select, from A to E, which one of the above is the generic name for:

Q48 Imodium C

Q49 Guttalax B · x Ⓓ ·

Q50 Senokot A

Questions 51–54: Match the lettered generic name most closely corresponding to the numbered proprietary (brand) name:

A ☐ sodium cromoglicate
B ☐ budesonide
C ☐ gentamicin
D ☐ mefenamic acid
E ☐ salbutamol

Select, from **A** to **E**, which one of the above is the generic name for:

Q51   Ponstan Forte   D

Q52   Ventolin   E

Q53   Pulmicort   B

Q54   Garamycin   C

Questions 55–58: Match the lettered dosage strength with its most closely corresponding numbered generic name:

A ☐ 20 mg
B ☐ 500 mg
C ☐ 5 mg
D ☐ 100 mg
E ☐ 75 mg

Select, from **A** to **E**, which one of the above dosages is used for:

Q55   atenolol tablets   D

Q56   prednisolone tablets   C

Q57   ranitidine tablets   E

Q58   paracetamol tablets   B

Questions 59–61 concern the following preparations:

A   ☐   ascorbic acid
B   ☐   acetylsalicylic acid
C   ☐   thiamine
D   ☐   acetaminophen
E   ☐   fluoride

Select, from A to E, which one of the above is the chemical name for:

Q59   aspirin   *B .*

Q60   paracetamol   *D .*

Q61   vitamin C   *A*

Questions 62–78

Directions: For each of the questions below, ONE or MORE of the responses is (are) correct. Decide which of the responses is (are) correct. Then choose:

A   ☐   if 1, 2 and 3 are correct
B   ☐   if 1 and 2 only are correct
C   ☐   if 2 and 3 only are correct
D   ☐   if 1 only is correct
E   ☐   if 3 only is correct

Directions summarised				
A	**B**	**C**	**D**	**E**
1, 2, 3	1, 2 only	2, 3 only	1 only	3 only

Q62 A patient with hypertension should be advised to avoid:

1 ☐ antihistamines
2 ☑ oral rehydration salts C
3 ☑ sympathomimetics

(E) ✗

Q63 Naproxen:

1 ☑ inhibits prostaglandin synthesis
D. 2 ☐ inhibits bradykinin release
3 ☐ increases body temperature

Q64 Naprosyn is available commercially as:

1 ☑ tablets
D 2 ☐ suppositories
3 ☐ capsules

Q65 Angiotensin-converting enzyme inhibitors should be used with caution in patients:

1 ☑ receiving diuretics
B 2 ☑ with renal disease
3 ☐ with hypertension

Q66 When dispensing glyceryl trinitrate tablets to a patient, they should be advised to:

1 ☑ discard tablets 8 weeks after opening
B 2 ☑ keep tablets in original container and keep tightly closed
3 ☐ chew tablets as necessary

Q67   The following drugs may precipitate an asthma attack:

1   ☑ beta-adrenoceptor blockers
2   ☑ non-steroidal anti-inflammatory drugs
3   ☐ paracetamol

B.

Q68   Which of the following agents is (are) indicated for the prophylaxis of migraine headache?

1   ☐ ergotamine
2   ☑ propranolol
3   ☑ amitriptyline

C

Q69   Medicines associated with anaphylactic shock include:

1   ☑ antibacterial agents
2   ☑ vaccines
3   ☐ NSAIDs

+B.

Q70   Ipratropium bromide:

1   ☑ is an antimuscarinic agent
2   ☐ is contraindicated in asthma patients
3   ☐ is only available as a solid oral dosage form

D

Q71   Acetazolamide:

1   ☑ may be used in the treatment of glaucoma
2   ☑ is a carbonic anhydrase inhibitor
3   ☐ is available as eye drops

A

Q72   Warfarin:

1   ☑ is available as 1, 3, 5 mg tablets
2   ☐ has hypersensitivity as the main adverse effect
3   ☐ price per tablet is about €2.5 (£1.60)

D

Q73 Chlorhexidine gluconate:

1   ☑ inhibits the formation of plaque on teeth
2   ☑ may cause teeth staining
3   ☑ is available as Corsodyl mouthwash

Q74 Antibacterial agents used topically in the treatment of acne include:

1   ☐ erythromycin
2   ☑ tetracycline
3   ☑ isotretinoin

Q75 Acid rebound is likely to occur with the chronic use of large doses of which of the following preparations?

1   ☐ aluminium hydroxide
2   ☐ magnesium hydroxide
3   ☑ calcium carbonate

Q76 Which of the following drugs would be effective in the treatment of Parkinson's disease?

1   ☐ co-careldopa
2   ☐ orphenadrine
3   ☐ trifluoperazine

Q77 Metronidazole:

1   ☐ is an antifungal agent
2   ☐ is active against protozoa
3   ☑ causes disulfiram-like reaction with alcohol

Q78 For the treatment of corns and calluses:

1   ☐ salicylic acid is used as a keratolytic
2   ☐ epidermabrasion is a safe method of treatment
3   ☐ imidazole antifungals may be recommended

Questions 79–82

Directions: The following questions consist of a first statement followed by a second statement. Decide whether the first statement is true or false. Decide whether the second statement is true or false. Then choose:

A   ☐   if both statements are true and the second statement is a *correct explanation* of the first statement

B   ☐   if both statements are true but the second statement *is NOT a correct explanation* of the first statement

C   ☐   if the first statement is true but the second statement is false

D   ☐   if the first statement is false but the second statement is true

E   ☐   if both statements are false

Directions summarised			
	First statement	**Second statement**	
A	True	True	Second statement is a *correct explanation* of the first
B	True	True	Second statement is *NOT a correct explanation* of the first
C	True	False	
D	False	True	
E	False	False	

Q79 Imodium can be used in children over 3 months. Imodium is an adsorbent drug.   D. Ⓔ ✗

Q80 Tardive dyskinesia is a chronic movement disorder characterised by uncontrolled facial movements. Tardive dyskinesia is associated with the use of trifluoperazine.   B.

Q81   Beclometasone (beclomethasone) dipropionate aerosol is used in the acute asthmatic attack. When used in conjunction with a bronchodilator administered by inhalation, the bronchodilator should be used first. D

Q82   Diuretic therapy is interrupted for 1 month when ACE inhibitors are being added to a patient's drug therapy. Diuretics interfere with the action of ACE inhibitors.   F   C

x (E)

Questions 83–100

Directions: These questions involve cases. Read the prescription or case and answer the questions.

Questions 83–87: Use the prescription below:

Patient's name   ....

Age   34 years

Klaricid 250 mg tabs
b.d.   m. 10
Codipront syrup
10 mL b.d.   m. 1 bottle

Doctor's signature   ....

Q83   The Codipront syrup prescribed is a combination product that contains an:

A   ☐ expectorant and an antitussive
B   ☐ expectorant and an antihistamine
C   ☐ antitussive and a nasal decongestant
D   ☑ antitussive and an antihistamine
E   ☐ expectorant and a nasal decongestant

Q84 The Klaricid product is:

A ☒ a macrolide, clarithromycin
B ☐ a macrolide, azithromycin
C ☐ a cephalosporin, cefuroxime axetil
D ☒ a cephalosporin, cefalexin
E ☐ a tetracycline, doxycycline

Q85 The patient develops vaginal thrush superinfection. The most appropriate treatment is:

A ☐ povidone-iodine
B ☐ clindamycin
C ☒ econazole
D ☐ sulphonamide
E ☐ penicillins

Q86 Which of the following have to be avoided when the patient is taking Klaricid?

A ☐ Burinex
B ☒ warfarin
C ☒ cimetidine
D ☐ naproxen
E ☐ phenylephrine

Q87 Which of the following auxiliary labels should be used during dispensing?

1 ☐ 'May cause drowsiness. If affected do not drive or operate machinery'
2 ☐ 'Take at regular intervals. Complete the prescribed course unless otherwise directed'
3 ☐ 'Avoid exposure of skin to direct sunlight or sunlamps'

A ☐ 1, 2, 3
B ☐ 1, 2 only
C ☐ 2, 3 only
D ☐ 1 only
E ☐ 3 only

Questions 88–91: Use the prescription below:

Patient's name   ....

Age   45 years

Prempak-C 0.0625 mg
1 daily
repeat for 3 months

Doctor's signature   ....

Q88 The active ingredient(s) in Prempak-C is (are):

A ☐ conjugated oestrogens
B ☒ conjugated oestrogens and norgestrel
C ☐ ethinylestradiol
D ☑ ethinylestradiol and levonorgestrel
E ☐ ethinylestradiol and gestodene

Q89 The patient is advised to:

1 ☐ have a 7-day interval between the three courses
C 2 ☑ take one tablet daily
3 ☑ start subsequent courses without interval

A ☐ 1, 2, 3
B ☐ 1, 2 only
C ☐ 2, 3 only
D ☐ 1 only
E ☐ 3 only

Q90 Absolute contraindications to the use of Prempak-C are:

1 ☑ thromboembolic disorders
2 ☑ oestrogen-dependent carcinoma
3 ☑ history of migraine

A ☐ 1, 2, 3
B ☐ 1, 2 only
C ☐ 2, 3 only
D ☐ 1 only
E ☐ 3 only

Q91 Other dosage forms available for the same line of treatment include:

1 ☐ self-adhesive patches
2 ☐ cream
3 ☐ pessaries

A ☐ 1, 2, 3
B ☐ 1, 2 only
C ☐ 2, 3 only
D ☐ 1 only
E ☐ 3 only

Questions 92–94: Use the case below:

A 24-year-old woman comes to the pharmacy with a new prescription for Tryptizol 25 mg tablets, two tablets t.d.s.

Q92 When dispensing the above prescription the pharmacist should advise the patient that side-effects to be expected are:

1   ☐ increased micturition
2   ☐ heartburn
3   ☐ drowsiness

A   ☐ 1, 2, 3
B   ☐ 1, 2 only
C   ☐ 2, 3 only
D   ☐ 1 only
E   ☐ 3 only

Q93 The label produced for the medicine dispensed to the patient should include:

A   ☐ take two tablets three times daily
B   ☐ take two tablets four times daily
C   ☑ take two tablets three times daily after meals
D   ☐ take two tablets three times daily before meals
E   ☐ take one tablet three times daily

Q94 The patient returns to the pharmacy after 4 days complaining that the drug is causing dry mouth, constipation and that the drug has not improved the symptoms of depression. The pharmacist should:

A ☐ tell the patient to stop taking the medication

B ☑ explain to the patient that these are expected side-effects of early treatment of the drug

C ☐ contact the prescriber that the drug is not effective in this patient

D ☐ contact the prescriber and report that the patient is suffering a hypersensitivity reaction to the drug

E ☐ inform the prescriber that an anticholinergic agent needs to be prescribed to this patient

Questions 95–96: Use the prescription below:

Patient's name	....
Age	21 years
Dalacin C 75 mg b.d. m. 180	
Doctor's signature	....

Q95 The patient states that they were prescribed for acne. The treatment duration is:

A ☑ at least 3 months

B ☐ not exceeding 3 days

C ☐ 5 days

D ☐ 2 weeks

E ☐ not exceeding 4 weeks

Q96   Dalacin C:

1   ☐ is a penicillin
2   ☐ is a broad-spectrum antibacterial agent
3   ☐ may cause antibiotic-associated colitis

A   ☐ 1, 2, 3
B   ☐ 1, 2 only
C   ☑ 2, 3 only
D   ☐ 1 only
E   ☒ 3 only

Questions 97–100: Use the prescription below:

Patient's name	....
Age	68 years
Euglucon 5 mg tabs o.m. m. 30	
Doctor's signature	....

Q97   Euglucon acts mainly by:

A   ☒ increasing insulin secretion
B   ☐ regulating carbohydrate metabolism
C   ☐ decreasing gluconeogenesis
D   ☑ increasing utilisation of glucose
E   ☐ delaying absorption of starch

Q98 Hypoglycaemia may develop if the patient:

1 ☐ skips meals
2 ☐ follows a weight-reducing diet
3 ☐ misses Euglucon tablets

b

A ☐ 1, 2, 3
B ☐ 1, 2 only
C ☐ 2, 3 only
D ☐ 1 only
E ☐ 3 only

Q99 Signs that indicate hypoglycaemia include:

1 ☐ nausea and vomiting
2 ☐ perspiration
3 ☐ palpitations

Ⓒ

D✗ A ☐ 1, 2, 3
B ☐ 1, 2 only
C ☐ 2, 3 only
D ☐ 1 only
E ☐ 3 only

Q100 The patient returns to the pharmacy complaining of very frequent attacks of hypoglycaemia, especially during the night. When contacted by the prescriber, which alternative treatment may be recommended:

A ☐ chlorpropamide
B ☐ acarbose
C ☑ gliclazide
D ☐ repaglinide
E ☐ insulin

Test 6

Answers

A1 D

Ammonium chloride is an expectorant similar to guaifenesin. Sedating anti-histamines, such as diphenhydramine, have antitussive properties. Dextromethorphan, pholcodine and codeine phosphate are opioid anti-tussives. Codeine tends to cause constipation whereas dextromethorphan and pholcodine have fewer side-effects. Codeine and pholcodine are more potent than dextromethorphan.

A2 B

When dispensing eye drops, patients are advised to tilt back their head, pull down the lower eyelid with the index finger and instil the drops without touching the eyelid with tip of the dropper. Patients are then advised to keep their eyes closed for 2–3 min. Any excess liquid drops can be wiped away from the face. The eye dropper is replaced and capped. Patients applying more than one type of eye drops are advised to allow an interval of 5 min between one medication and another.

A3 C

Benzoyl peroxide promotes the shedding of keratinised epithelial cells on the skin and is therefore a keratolytic agent. In the treatment of acne it is indicated as a first-line agent in the form of topical preparations. Benzoyl peroxide is mildly irritant, particularly during the early stages of treatment and hence a low strength is chosen to initiate treatment. Moreover aqueous preparations are preferred over alcoholic preparations, to avoid irritation.

A4 C

Naproxen is a non-steroidal anti-inflammatory agent classified as a propionic acid derivative.

A5 B

An amount of 5000 mg is equivalent to 5 g which is equivalent to 0.005 kg.

A6 E

The daily dose for a patient weighing 67 kg is 335 mg (67 × 5), meaning that the drug must be administered 112 mg three times daily (every 8 h).

A7 A

Ointments are given as w/w %. Therefore 1% hydrocortisone ointment is equivalent to 1 g of hydrocortisone per 100 g of ointment.

Hence:

$$0.5 \text{ g hydrocortisone per } 100 \text{ g ointment}$$
$$= ? \text{ g per } 30 \text{ g}$$
$$= (30 \text{ g} \times 0.5)/100 \text{ g}$$
$$= 0.15 \text{ g hydrocortisone in } 30 \text{ g ointment}$$

$$1 \text{ g hydrocortisone in } 100 \text{ g ointment}$$
$$= 0.15 \text{ g in } ? \text{ g hydrocortisone } 1\%$$
$$= 100 \text{ g} \times 0.15 \text{ g}$$
$$= 15 \text{ g hydrocortisone } 1\%$$

Therefore 15 g of the 1% hydrocortisone ointment need to be diluted with white soft paraffin to make up 30 g of 0.5% hydrocortisone ointment.

A8 C

Ondansetron is a $5HT_3$ antagonist indicated as an anti-emetic agent in nausea and vomiting associated with chemotherapy. The dose administered depends on the emetogenic degree of the chemotherapeutic agents used.

A9 B

Normal saline (0.9%) relieves nasal congestion by liquifying mucous secretions thereby acting as a nasal decongestant. It is safely recommended for use in infants. Topical administration of sympathomimetic nasal decongestants such as pseudoephedrine in infants may lead to irritation with narrowing of the nasal passages. Systemic use of the sympathomimetics increases the risk of side-effects, such as tachycardia, making systemic use of nasal decongestants all the more contraindicated in infants. Cetirizine is a non-sedating antihistamine. Antihistamines tend to be more effective in reducing rhinorrhoea and sneezing rather than nasal congestion. Mefenamic acid is a non-steroidal anti-inflammatory.

A10 C

Gentamicin is an aminoglycoside. All aminoglycosides tend to be nephrotoxic and ototoxic. The dose must be reduced and serum concentrations must be monitored in patients with nephrotoxicity. Concomitant administration of aminoglycosides and other nephrotoxic drugs, such as diuretics, cyclosporin, teicoplanin and vancomycin should be avoided.

A11 D

Salbutamol is a selective $beta_1$ agonist and therefore mimics the sympathetic system resulting in tachycardia and fine tremor. Salbutamol causes potassium loss leading to the development of muscle cramps. It also leads to headache. Constipation is not a side-effect of salbutamol but is commonly associated with the use of antimuscarinics.

A12   A

Bezafibrate is a lipid-regulating drug classified as a fibrate. Fibrates act by reducing the serum triglycerides and low-density lipoproteins (LDLs) and raising high-density lipoprotein (HDL) cholesterol levels. Statins, which inhibit the enzyme 3-hydroxy-3-methylglutaryl coenzyme A (HMG CoA), tend to be less effective than fibrates in reducing triglyceride levels and raising the HDL cholesterol levels but more effective than the fibrates in lowering LDL cholesterol levels.

A13   A

Otrivine is a proprietary (trade name) preparation of xylometazoline, a nasal decongestant. The maximum dose recommended is three drops into each nostril three to four times daily. The drops are not recommended for children under 2 years of age.

A14   A

Citalopram is a selective serotonin re-uptake inhibitor (SSRI). These tend to have fewer antimuscarinic effects than tricyclic antidepressant (TCA) drugs, such as dry mouth and constipation; however, SSRIs tend to cause gastrointestinal effects, such as nausea and vomiting. MAOIs are monoamine oxidase inhibitors.

A15   C

Dioralyte is a proprietary preparation of oral rehydration salts containing electrolytes, namely sodium chloride, potassium chloride, sodium bicarbonate, citric acid and glucose. Picolax and Citramag are proprietary preparations classified as bowel-cleansing solutions used before gastrointestinal examination procedures, to ensure that the bowel is free of solid material. Ensure is a nutritional supplement. Kay-Cee-L is a preparation containing potassium chloride, which is indicated in potassium depletion.

A16   B

Fucicort contains fusidic acid (antibacterial) and betamethasone (a potent corticosteroid). Eurax cream contains the antihistamine crotamiton, Dermovate preparations contain the potent corticosteroid clobetasol, Nerisone preparations contain the potent corticosteroid diflucortolone and Pevaryl preparations contain the imidazole antifungal econazole.

A17   A

The recommended dose of paracetamol for a 5-year-old child is 250 mg every 4–6 h.

A18   A

Levonorgestrel is a progestogen derivative. It is found either in combined oral contraceptives coupled with an oestrogen derivative or alone in progestogen-only contraceptives.

A19   A

Aciclovir is an antiviral indicated in the treatment and prophylaxis of cold sores. It is available for systemic administration (tablets) or topical use (cream, eye ointment). In the management of cold sores, the cream is applied every 4 h and continued for 5 days. Its use should be started as soon as symptoms (tingling sensation) begin.

A20   B

Carbimazole is an antithyroid drug indicated in hyperthyroidism. It is usually administered as 15 mg daily in the morning. Carbimazole tends to cause agranulocytosis and therefore patients are advised to report immediately any signs of infections, such as sore throat.

A21   B

Desloratadine is a non-sedating antihistamine. Diphenhydramine, chlor-phenamine (chlorpheniramine), promethazine and alimemazine (trimeprazine) are sedating antihistamines with diphenhydramine and promethazine being marketed in over-the-counter hypnotic preparations.

A22   C

Alginic acid tends to prevent gastro-oesophageal reflux. The antifoaming agent intended to relieve flatulence is dimeticone (simethicone).

A23   C

Parenteral preparations in the form of a suspension cannot be administered through the intravenous route. Preparations intended for administration in this way must be soluble solutions to avoid occlusion of the veins.

A24   A

Activated dimeticone (simethicone) is an antifoaming agent, which relieves flatulence and is used in infant colic.

A25   C

Gentamicin is an aminoglycoside. As aminoglycosides are not absorbed from the gastrointestinal tract, gentamicin is only presented for parenteral or topical use (as eye/ear drops).

A26   B

Tinea pedis is a fungal infection commonly known as athlete's foot. Chickenpox is a childhood infection caused by the herpes zoster virus.

Hepatitis is a viral infection of the liver. Mumps is a viral infection characterised by bilateral or unilateral inflammation of the salivary glands. Rubella (German measles) is caused by the rubella virus.

A27   E

Sunscreen preparations with a sun protection factor of eight allow people to stay in the sun without burning eight times longer than those not using any sun protection factor. The higher the factor the greater the degree of protection.

A28   B

Bioavailability is defined as the relative amount of drug that reaches the systemic circulation and the rate at which the drug appears in the circulation.

A29   B

Disintegration into fine particles is the first process that occurs when a drug is administered as a solid dosage form. The effectiveness of a tablet or solid dosage form in releasing the drug depends on the rate of disintegration. Dissolution rate is the rate at which the solid fine particle dissolves in a solvent.

A30   A

Lorazepam is a short-acting benzodiazepine indicated for use in relieving anxiety and insomnia. Lorazepam may also be administered peri-operatively to alleviate pain and in status epilepticus. Imipramine is a tricyclic antidepressant, paroxetine is a selective serotonin re-uptake inhibitor, venlafaxine is a serotonin and adrenaline (epinephrine) re-uptake inhibitor and moclobemide is a reversible monoamine oxidase inhibitor. Imipramine, paroxetine, venlafaxine and moclobemide are all classified as antidepressants.

A31 C

Common childhood vaccines include the three-in-one measles, mumps and rubella and the diphtheria vaccine. Infectious mononucleosis, also known as glandular fever, is caused by the Epstein-Barr virus and no vaccine is available.

A32 C

The rubella virus results in a self-limiting infection characterised by a rash spreading from the face, trunk and limbs. The infection commonly occurs in children. The rubella virus has the most serious effect on the fetus. Rubella occurring during pregnancy, especially during the first trimester, may result in spontaneous abortion, stillbirths or congenital malformations.

A33 D

The first-line agents in the treatment of rheumatoid arthritis are non-steroidal anti-inflammatory drugs such as diclofenac. Diclofenac and indometacin, another NSAID, tend to have similar activity; however, indometacin has a higher incidence of side-effects and therefore diclofenac is more appropriate for initial treatment. Sodium aurothiomalate is classified as a disease-modifying antirheumatic drug and is used as second-line treatment in rheumatoid arthritis. Paracetamol is often indicated in the management of osteoarthritis. Local intra-articular injections of dexamethasone may be administered for the relief of soft-tissue inflammatory conditions.

A34 C

Patients allergic to penicillin may be cross-sensitive to cephalosporins. Cephalosporins (cefaclor, first-generation cephalosporin) are therefore avoided in these patients and instead macrolides (for example, erythromycin) are generally administered. Ketoconazole is an imidazole antifungal agent.

A35 D

Meloxicam is a partially selective cyclo-oxygenase-2 inhibitor and is therefore less likely to cause gastrointestinal side-effects, such as bleeding, than other NSAIDs.

A36 C

Paracetamol overdose is most likely to cause hepatic necrosis and to a lesser extent renal necrosis. Hepatic necrosis is maximal within 3–4 h of ingestion and may lead to encephalopathy, haemorrhage, hypoglycaemia, cerebral oedema and death. Acetylcysteine tends to protect the liver if given within 10–12 h of paracetamol poisoning. The maximum adult dose of paracetamol is 4 g in 24 h.

A37 B

Diazepam (benzodiazepine) is indicated for the treatment of status epilepticus (prolonged febrile convulsions) when it is administered intravenously or rectally. Lorazepam (benzodiazepine), which has a longer duration of action, could also be used in status epilepticus.

A38 A

Hydrocortisone is available orally. Other corticosteroids also available orally include prednisolone, betamethasone, cortisone acetate, deflazacort, methylprednisolone, dexamethasone and fluocortolone.

A39 A

Hydrocortisone is the least potent corticosteroid.

A40 D

Fluticasone is available for inhalation as Flixotide inhaler or Flixonase nasal spray.

A41 A

Furosemide (frusemide), a loop diuretic, inhibits re-absorption from the ascending loop of Henle in the renal tubule.

A42 A

Loop diuretics should be used with caution in patients with urinary retention, for example, patients with enlarged prostrate as they may cause urinary retention. Small doses and less potent diuretics should be used.

A43 C

Spironolactone is a potassium-sparing diuretic. It is an aldosterone antagonist and potentiates the action of loop or thiazide diuretics.

A44 A

Chlorpromazine is an aliphatic antipsychotic with marked sedative properties.

A45 D

Thioridazine is an antipsychotic classified as a piperadine. Thioridazine is associated with a lower incidence of extrapyramidal effects compared with other antipsychotics. However, thioridazine may be associated with antimuscarinic effects and sedation.

A46   B

Flupentixol is an antipsychotic classified as a thioxanthene. Thioxanthenes have pronounced extrapyramidal side-effects.

A47   A

Largactil is a proprietary preparation of chlorpromazine.

A48   C

Imodium is a proprietary preparation of loperamide used as an antidiarrhoeal.

A49   D

Guttalax is a proprietary preparation of sodium picosulfate. Sodium picosulfate is a stimulant laxative that increases intestinal motility.

A50   A

Senokot is a proprietary preparation of senna, a stimulant laxative. Stimulant laxatives increase intestinal motility and act in a relatively short time.

A51   D

Ponstan Forte is a proprietary preparation of mefenamic acid, a non-steroidal anti-inflammatory drug.

A52   E

Ventolin is a proprietary preparation of salbutamol, a selective $beta_2$ agonist indicated as a reliever in asthma.

A53   B

Pulmicort is a proprietary preparation of budesonide, a corticosteroid inhaler indicated as a prophylactic agent in asthma.

A54   C

Garamycin is a proprietary preparation of the aminoglycoside gentamicin. Garamycin is available as ear/eye drops.

A55   D

Atenolol (water soluble beta-adrenoceptor blocker) is available as 25 mg, 50 mg or 100 mg tablets.

A56   C

Prednisolone (corticosteroid) is available as 1 mg, 2.5 mg, 5 mg and 25 mg tablets.

A57   E

Ranitidine (H_2-receptor antagonist) is available as 75 mg, 150 mg and 300 mg tablets.

A58   B

Paracetamol is available as 500 mg tablets.

A59   B

Acetylsalicylic acid is the chemical name for aspirin.

A60 D

Acetaminophen is the chemical name for paracetamol.

A61 A

Ascorbic acid is the chemical name for vitamin C.

A62 E

Sympathomimetics mimic the sympathetic system thereby increasing the force of contraction of the heart and the blood pressure. Sympathomimetics are therefore contraindicated in patients with hypertension.

A63 D

Naproxen, a non-steroidal anti-inflammatory drug, inhibits prostaglandin release through inhibition of the cyclo-oxygenase-2 enzyme, producing an analgesic and anti-inflammatory effect.

A64 D

Naprosyn (naproxen, a non-steroidal anti-inflammatory drug) is available as tablets.

A65 B

Angiotensin-converting enzyme inhibitors should be used with caution in patients taking diuretics because of an enhanced hypotensive effect. Angiotensin-converting enzyme inhibitors should also be used with caution in patients with renal impairment. Renal function needs to be monitored in patients with renovascular disease.

A66   B

Patients using sublingual glyceryl trinitrate tablets are advised to take a tablet at the first sign of angina. Patients can take three sublingual tablets in 15 minutes after which they must seek professional advice. Patients are advised to keep the tablets handy and in the original container because of instability. The tablets should be dissolved sublingually and not chewed. The tablets must be discarded 8 weeks after opening.

A67   B

Beta-adrenoceptor blockers block the sympathetic system antagonising the effect on the lungs, resulting in bronchoconstriction. Non-steroidal anti-inflammatory drugs inhibit prostaglandin synthesis, which may lead to bronchoconstriction.

A68   C

Ergotamine is an ergot alkaloid derivative indicated in the treatment of migraine. Propranolol (fat-soluble beta-blocker) and amitriptyline (tricyclic antidepressant) are used for the prophylaxis of migraine headache.

A69   A

Antibacterial agents, vaccines and non-steroidal anti-inflammatory drugs (NSAIDs) may all lead to anaphylactic shock if the patient is allergic to these medicines.

A70   D

Ipratropium bromide is an antimuscarinic agent indicated in asthma and in chronic obstructive pulmonary disease but it is more effective in the latter. The drug is available only for inhalation because of the potential side-effects if given orally.

A71   B

Acetazolamide is a carbonic anhydrase inhibitor, which reduces intra-ocular pressure by reducing aqueous humour production. It is used in the treatment of glaucoma. Acetazolamide is administered systemically. Recently newer carbonic anhydrase inhibitors have been developed, which are available as topical agents (for example, dorzolamide).

A72   D

Warfarin is an oral anticoagulant agent available as 1 mg (brown tablets), 3 mg (blue tablets) and 5 mg (pink tablets). The main side-effect of warfarin is increased bleeding. The approximate price of warfarin per tablet is €0.02 (£0.013).

A73   A

Chlorhexidine gluconate inhibits the formation of plaque on teeth and is indicated in oral infections and periodontal disease. Chlorhexidine gluconate is available as Corsodyl mouthwash. Long-term use of chlorhexidine may result in staining of the teeth.

A74   B

Antibacterial preparations that may be used topically in acne include erythromycin, tetracycline and clindamycin. Isotretinoin is a tretinoin isomer used in the management of acne.

A75   E

Antacids containing calcium carbonate have the greatest neutralising capacity but tend to cause acid rebound with long-term use. Calcium carbonate may also lead to hypercalcaemia and the milk-alkali syndrome which is characterised by nausea, headache and renal damage.

A76   B

Co-careldopa is a combination of levodopa and the peripheral dopa-decarboxylase inhibitor. Co-careldopa is indicated in Parkinson's disease to improve bradykinesia and rigidity rather than tremor. Orphenadrine is an antimuscarinic agent indicated in patients with Parkinson's disease where tremor predominates. Trifluoperazine is a piperazine antipsychotic which should be used with caution in patients with Parkinson's disease as its use may exacerbate the condition.

A77   C

Metronidazole is an antiprotozoal agent which, if taken concomitantly with alcohol, may result in a disulfiram-like reaction characterised by intense vasodilation, headache, tachycardia, sweating and vomiting.

A78   B

Salicylic acid is a keratolytic agent that removes layers of cornified skin cells. Treatment for corns, calluses and warts involves the application of salicylic acid at a concentration of 11–50%. Salicylic acid is contraindicated in allergic patients and its use should be avoided in diabetic patients. Epidermabrasion refers to the physical process of removing the horny skin layer using a mechanical aid. It does not involve any pharmacological agents and is a safe and effective method for removing corns and calluses. Corns and calluses occurring in diabetic patients should be managed with care as diabetic patients may have a compromised peripheral circulation.

A79   E

Imodium is a proprietary preparation of loperamide, an antidiarrhoeal drug indicated for use in adults and children over 12 years. Loperamide should not be administered in children under 4 years who have diarrhoea. Children are more sensitive to the occurrence of respiratory depression. Fluid and electrolyte replacement are first-line treatments in diarrhoea.

A80   B

Tardive dyskinesia is a chronic movement disorder characterised by uncontrolled facial movement disorders. Tardive dyskinesia is associated with the use of antipsychotics such as trifluoperazine.

A81   D

Beclometasone (beclomethasone) dipropionate aerosol inhaler is a corticosteroid. Corticosteroids are used as prophylaxis in patients with asthma and therefore have no use in an acute attack. Bronchodilators acting as relievers are indicated for an acute attack. In asthma, patients are advised first to administer the bronchodilator, which acts very fast and then apply the corticosteroid, which has anti-inflammatory properties.

A82   E

Concomitant administration of diuretics and angiotensin-converting enzyme (ACE) inhibitors results in enhanced hypotensive effect. Blood pressure monitoring is required, therefore, if patients who are on diuretics are started on ACE inhibitors, the ACE inhibitor should be initiated in the evening to avoid falls due to hypotension.

A83   D

Codipront syrup contains codeine, an antitussive and phenyltoloxamine, an antihistamine. The combination is indicated for dry cough.

A84 A

Klaricid is a proprietary preparation of the macrolide, clarithromycin. Clarithromycin tends to be more effective against Gram-positive agents when compared with erythromycin. Clarithromycin 250 mg is administered twice daily whereas clarithromycin 500 mg is administered once daily.

A85 C

The use of imidazole antifungal agents such as econazole is the mainstay of treatment in vaginal thrush (candidiasis).

A86 B

When administered concomitantly, clarithromycin and the oral anticoagulant warfarin may interact, resulting in an enhanced anticoagulant effect and therefore increased risk of bleeding.

A87 B

Codipront may cause drowsiness because of the antihistamine component phenyltoloxamine and patients should be advised to avoid operating machinery and driving. Patients taking antibiotics should be advised to take the medicines at regular intervals and to complete the course of treatment prescribed.

A88 B

Prempak-C contains conjugated oestrogens and the progestogen component norgestrel. The combination is indicated as hormone replacement therapy in women with a uterus. Women who have undergone hysterectomy need the conjugated oestrogens component only.

A89   C

Patients on hormone replacement therapy such as Prempak-C are advised to take one tablet daily, starting subsequent courses without interval.

A90   B

Prempak-C is contraindicated in oestrogen-dependent carcinoma and thromboembolic disorders. A history of migraine is not an absolute contraindication but requires administration with caution. Migraine is a side-effect associated with the oestrogen component.

A91   B

Hormone replacement therapy is also available as self-adhesive patches and creams.

A92   E

Tryptizol is a proprietary preparation of the tricylic antidepressant amitriptyline. Tricylic antidepressants tend to have antimuscarinic side-effects, such as urinary retention, blurred vision, dry mouth and sweating. They also tend to cause drowsiness.

A93   A

In this case the patient is advised to take two tablets three times daily.

A94   B

Tricylic antidepressants such as amitriptyline (Tryptizol) cause antimuscarinic side-effects, such as dry mouth and constipation. These antidepressants also tend to exhibit a time lag of about 3 weeks before the symptoms of depression are improved. Patients must be advised about the potential side-effects and that the drug may take some time to have an effect.

A95   A

Treatment for acne usually takes at least 3 months. In this case the patient must take one Dalacin C tablet twice daily for 3 months.

A96   E

Dalacin C contains the antimicrobial clindamycin, which is active against Gram-positive organisms and may cause antibiotic-associated colitis.

A97   A

Euglucon is an oral antidiabetic agent containing the sulphonylurea gliben-clamide. It acts by increasing insulin secretion and is therefore indicated in type 2 diabetes (non-insulin dependent) where there is pancreatic activity.

A98   B

Hypoglycaemic attacks may develop if the patient follows weight-reducing diets and skips meals. The patient is therefore advised to carry sweets, to be eaten if signs of hypoglycaemia develop.

A99   C

Signs characteristic of hypoglycaemia include sweating, palpitations, pallor, tremor and weakness.

A100   C

Glibenclamide is a long-acting sulphonylurea and therefore may result in hypo-glycaemic attacks, especially during the night. Gliclazide is a short-acting sulphonylurea, consequently presenting a lower risk of hypoglycaemic attacks.

Bibliography

Azzopardi LM (2000). *Validation Instruments for Community Pharmacy: Pharmaceutical Care for the Third Millennium*. Binghamton, New York: Pharmaceutical Products Press.

Como DN (1998). *Mosby's Medical, Nursing and Allied Health Dictionary*, 5th edn. St Louis, Missouri: Mosby.

Edwards C, Stillman P (2000). *Minor Illness or Major Disease? Responding to Symptoms in the Pharmacy*, 3rd edn. London: Pharmaceutical Press.

Greene RJ, Harris ND (2000). *Pathology and Therapeutics for Pharmacists: a Basis for Clinical Pharmacy Practice*, 2nd edn. London: Pharmaceutical Press.

Hardman JG, Limbird LE, Goodman Gilman A (2001). *Goodman & Gilman's The Pharmacological Basis of Therapeutics*, 10th edn. New York: McGraw-Hill.

Harman RJ, ed (2000). *Handbook of Pharmacy Health-Education*, 2nd edn. London: Pharmaceutical Press.

Harman RJ, Mason P, eds (2002). *Handbook of Pharmacy Healthcare: Diseases and Patient Advice*, 2nd edn. London: Pharmaceutical Press.

Mehta DK, ed (2002). *British National Formulary*, 44th edn. London: Pharmaceutical Press.

Nathan A (2002). *Non-prescription Medicines*, 2nd edn. London: Pharmaceutical Press.

Pagana KD, Pagana TJ (1998). *Mosby's Manual of Diagnostic and Laboratory Tests*. St Louis, Missouri: Mosby.

Medicines, Ethics and Practice: a Guide for Pharmacists, 26 July 2002. London: Royal Pharmaceutical Society of Great Britain, 2002.

Sweetman SC, ed (2002). *Martindale: the Complete Drug Reference*, 33rd edn. London: Pharmaceutical Press.

Taylor LM (2002). *Pharmacy Preregistration Handbook: A Survival Guide*, 2nd edn. London: Pharmaceutical Press.

Appendix A

Proprietary (trade) names and equivalent generic names

The proprietary names used in this book can be found in Martindale: the Complete Drug Reference, *although not all are listed in the* British National Formulary.

ACT-HIB	*Haemophilus influenzae* type b vaccine
Actifed	triprolidine, pseudoephedrine
Actifed Compound Linctus	triprolidine, pseudoephedrine, dextromethorphan
Adalat	nifedipine
Aldactone	spironolactone
Alka-Seltzer	aspirin, citric acid, sodium bicarbonate
Alupent	orciprenaline
Amoxil	amoxicillin
Anacal	heparinoid, laureth '9'
Anadin	aspirin, caffeine
Anadin Extra	aspirin, paracetamol, caffeine
Anthisan	mepyramine
Anusol	bismuth, Peru balsam, zinc oxide
Arcalion	sulbutiamine
Arthrotec	diclofenac, misoprostol
Aspro	aspirin
Ativan	lorazepam
Augmentin	co-amoxiclav (amoxicillin, clavulanic acid)
Avomine	promethazine
Bactroban	mupirocin
Beconase	beclometasone (beclomethasone)
Beechams Hot Lemon and Honey	paracetamol, ascorbic acid, phenylephrine
Benzamycin	benzoyl peroxide, erythromycin
Betadine	povidone-iodine
Betnovate	betamethasone
Biodramina	dimenhydrinate

Bradosol	benzalkonium
Bricanyl	terbutaline
Bronchathiol	carbocisteine
BurnEze	benzocaine
Buscopan	hyoscine butylbromide
Buspar	buspirone
Ca-C	calcium, vitamin C
Canesten	clotrimazole
Canesten HC	clotrimazole, hydrocortisone
Cardura	doxazosin
Cerumol	arachis oil, paradichlorobenzene, chlorobutanol
Cilest	ethinylestradiol, norgestimate
Ciprobay	ciprofloxacin
Cirrus	cetirizine, pseudoephedrine
Citramag	magnesium carbonate, citric acid
Clarinase	loratidine, pseudoephedrine
Clarityn	loratidine
Codipront	codeine, phenyltoloxamine
Codipront cum Expectorans	codeine, guaifenesin, phenyltoloxamine
Codis	aspirin, codeine
Colofac	mebeverine
Conotrane	benzalkonium, dimeticone
Contac 400	phenylpropanolamine, chlorphenamine (chlorpheniramine)
Corsodyl	chlorhexidine
Cozaar	losartan
Cymalon	sodium citrate
Cytotec	misoprostol
Daktacort	miconazole, hydrocortisone
Daktarin	miconazole
Dalacin C	clindamycin
Dalacin T	clindamycin
Day Nurse	paracetamol, phenylpropanolamine, dextromethorphan
Deltacortril	prednisolone
Dequacaine	dequalinium, benzocaine
Dermovate	clobetasol
Dexa-Rhinaspray Duo	dexamethasone, tramazoline

Diamox	acetazolamide
Difflam	benzydamine
Diflucan	fluconazole
Dioralyte	sodium chloride, sodium bicarbonate, potassium chloride, citric acid, glucose
Distaclor	cefaclor
Distalgesic	paracetamol, dextropropoxyphene
Dovonex	calcipotriol
Dristan	spray: oxymetazoline; tablets: aspirin, chlorphenamine (chlorpheniramine), phenylephrine
Dulcolax	bisacodyl
Duphalac	lactulose
Dyspamet	cimetidine
E45	light liquid paraffin, white soft paraffin, hypoallergenic hydrous wool fat (lanolin)
Engerix B	hepatitis B surface antigen
Ensure	nutritional supplement
Erythroped	erythromycin
Euglucon	glibenclamide
Eurax	crotamiton
Fefol	iron, folic acid
Feldene	piroxicam
Fluarix	influenza vaccine
Forceval	multivitamin preparation containing vitamins and minerals
Fucicort	fusidic acid, betamethasone
Fucidin	fusidic acid
Fucidin H	fusidic acid, hydrocortisone
Fucithalmic	fusidic acid
Fulcin	griseofulvin
Fybogel	ispaghula husk
Garamycin	gentamicin
Gaviscon	oral suspension: calcium carbonate, alginate, sodium bicarbonate; tablets: alginic acid, aluminium hydroxide, magnesium trisilicate, sodium bicarbonate
Guttalax	sodium picosulfate
Gyno-Daktarin	miconazole

Havrix	formaldehyde-inactivated hepatitis A virus
Heminevrin	clomethiazole
Histergan	diphenhydramine
Hydrocortisyl	hydrocortisone
Imodium	loperamide
Inderal	propranolol
Indocid	indometacin
Irfen	ibuprofen
Isordil	isosorbide dinitrate
Istin	amlodipine
Karvol	levomenthol, chlorobutanol, pine oils, terpineol, thymol
Kay-Cee-L	potassium chloride
Klaricid	clarithromycin
Lamisil	terbinafine
Lanoxin	digoxin
Largactil	chlorpromazine
Lasix	furosemide (frusemide)
Lescol	fluvastatin
Lexomil	bromazepam
Lipobase	fatty cream base
Livial	tibolone
Livostin	levocabastine
Locabiotal	fusafungine
Locoid	hydrocortisone butyrate
Locorten-Vioform	clioquinol, flumetasone
Logynon	ethinylestradiol, levonorgestrel
Lomotil	diphenoxylate, atropine
Losec	omeprazole
Ludiomil	maprotiline
Maalox	aluminium hydroxide, magnesium hydroxide
Meggezones	menthol
Microgynon	ethinylestradiol, levonorgestrel
Mictral	nalidixic acid
Migraleve	codeine, buclizine, paracetamol
Migril	ergotamine, cyclizine, caffeine
Milk of Magnesia	magnesium hydroxide

Miocamen	midecamycin
Mobic	meloxicam
Mogadon	nitrazepam
Molcer	docusate sodium
Motilium	domperidone
Mucosolvan	ambroxol
Naprosyn	naproxen
Natrilix	indapamide
Nerisone	diflucortolone
Neurorubine-forte	vitamin B_1, B_6, B_{12}
Night Nurse	paracetamol, dextromethorphan, promethazine
Nootropil	piracetam
Noroxin	norfloxacin
Nupercainal	cinchocaine
Nu-Seals	aspirin
Oilatum	light liquid paraffin, white soft paraffin
Optrex	witch hazel
Orovite	vitamin B substances, vitamin C
Ortho-Gynest	estriol
Oruvail	ketoprofen
Otosporin	neomycin, polymyxin B, hydrocortisone
Otrisal	sodium chloride
Otrivine	xylometazoline
Panadol	paracetamol
Panadol Extra	paracetamol, caffeine
Pariet	rabeprazole
Pevaryl	econazole
Phenergan	promethazine
Picolax	sodium picosulfate, magnesium citrate
Polaramine	dexchlorpheniramine
Ponstan Forte	mefenamic acid
Ponstyl	mefenamic acid
Premarin	conjugated oestrogens
Prempak-C	conjugated oestrogens, norgestrel
Preparation H	shark liver oil, yeast cell extract
Proctosedyl	cinchocaine, hydrocortisone

Pulmicort	budesonide
Relifex	nabumetone
Rennie	calcium carbonate, magnesium carbonate
Rhinocap	phenylephrine, dimenhydrinate, caffeine
Rhinocort Aqua	budesonide
Rhinopront	phenylephrine, carbinoxamine
Rinstead	menthol, cetylpyridinium
Rulid	roxithromycin
Scholl Athlete's foot cream/spray	tolnaftate
Selenium-ACE	selenium, vitamins A, C, E
Senokot	sennosides
Serenace	haloperidol
Setlers Wind-eze	dimeticone
Silomat	clobutinol
Slow-K	potassium chloride
Slow-Fe Folic	iron, folic acid
Soframycin	framycetin
Solarcaine	lidocaine (lignocaine)
Solpadeine	paracetamol, codeine, caffeine
Spersallerg	antazoline, tetryzoline
Spersanicol	chloramphenicol
Stemetil	prochlorperazine
Stilnoct	zolpidem
Stugeron	cinnarizine
Sudocrem	benzyl alcohol, benzyl benzoate, benzyl cinnamate, lanolin, zinc oxide
Synalar	fluocinolone
Syndol	paracetamol, codeine, caffeine, doxylamine
Systral	chlorphenoxamine
Tagamet	cimetidine
Tegretol	carbamazepine
Telfast	fexofenadine
Tenormin	atenolol
Tildiem	diltiazem
Timoptol	timolol
Tinaderm	tolnaftate

Tramal	tramadol
Travocort	isoconazole, diflucortolone
Tryptizol	amitriptyline
Twinrix	inactivated hepatitis A virus, hepatitis B surface antigen
Uniflu	paracetamol, diphenydramine, phenylephrine, codeine, caffeine, ascorbic acid
Valium	diazepam
Vasogen	dimeticone, calamine, zinc oxide
Ventolin	salbutamol
Vermox	mebendazole
Viagra	sildenafil
Vioxx	rofecoxib
Voltarol	diclofenac
WaspEze	benzocaine, mepyramine
Waxsol	docusate sodium
Xalatan	latanoprost
Xanax	alprazolam
Xenical	orlistat
Xylocaine	lidocaine (lignocaine)
Xyloproct	lidocaine (lignocaine), hydrocortisone, aluminium acetate, zinc oxide
Xyzal	levocetirizine
Zaditen	ketotifen
Zantac	ranitidine
Zestril	lisinopril
Zinnat	cefuroxime
Zithromax	azithromycin
Zocor	simvastatin
Zofran	ondansetron
Zovirax	aciclovir

Appendix B

Definitions of conditions

Acne: skin disease occurring in the presence of sebaceous glands

Agranulocytosis: a drastic reduction in the white blood cell count

Allergic rhinitis: hay fever, inflammation of the nasal pathways

Alopecia: hair loss

Amenorrhoea: absence of menstruation

Angina: thoracic pain due to lack of oxygen supply to the myocardium

Anorexia: loss of appetite

Aphthous ulceration: canker sores, mouth sores

Arrhythmias: deviation in the pattern of heartbeat

Arthritis: inflammatory condition of the joints

Ascites: accumulation of fluid in the abdomen

Asthenia: loss of energy

Ataxia: inability to coordinate movements

Blepharitis: inflammation of the hair follicles and the meibomian glands of the eyelids

Bradycardia: heart rate less than 60 beats/min

Bronchodilatation: widening of the bronchi

Bulimia: food craving with overeating followed by purging

Calluses: hard skin occurring in areas prone to pressure or friction

Candidiasis: infection caused by *Candida* species

Cardiotoxicity: toxic effect to the cardiac tissues

Cataract: loss of transparency of the lens of the eye

Chilblains: areas of the skin that are inflamed and present as bluish-red in colour

Chloasma: skin pigmentation of the face occurring during pregnancy or with the use of oral contraceptives

Cholestatis: blocking of the bile pathway in the biliary system

Coeliac disease: inability to metabolise gluten

Cold sores: infection caused by herpes simplex virus

Conjunctivitis: inflammation of the conjunctiva

Contact dermatitis: skin irritation resulting from exposure to a sensitising antigen

Corns: mass of epithelial cells occurring over a bony prominence

Cradle cap: seborrhoeic dermatitis of the scalp occurring in infants

Crohn's disease: inflammatory disease of the gastrointestinal tract

Croup: viral infection of the upper respiratory tract occurring in infants

Cystitis: urinary tract bacterial infection

Dermatitis: inflammation of the skin

Diverticular disease: inflammation of diverticula

Ductus arteriosus: an opening in the fetal heart, which normally closes after birth, joining the pulmonary artery to the aorta

Dyspepsia: epigastric discomfort

Dysphagia: difficulty in swallowing

Dyspnoea: distress in breathing

Dysuria: painful urination

Eczema: skin dermatitis of unknown aetiology

Endometriosis: a condition characterised by growth of endometrial tissue outside the endometrium

Epidural analgesia: anaesthetic injected into the epidural space

Erythema: skin inflammation

Furuncles: boil, staphylococcal infection of a gland or hair follicle

Gastroenteritis: inflammatory condition of the stomach

Gingival hyperplasia: gum tissue overgrowth

Glaucoma: a raised intraocular pressure

Gout: increased uric acid resulting in sodium urate crystals deposited in the joints

Gynaecomastia: enlargement of one or both breasts in male

Haemorrhoids: varicosity in the lower gastrointestinal tract, specifically the rectum or anus

Heart failure: heart does not meet the requirements of the body and the pumping action is less than required

Hiatus hernia: protrusion of a portion of the stomach into the thorax through the oesophageal hiatus of the diaphragm

Hirsutism: excessive body hair in a masculine pattern

Hypercalcaemia: increased calcium blood level

Hyperglycaemia: high blood glucose level

Hyperhidrosis: increased perspiration

Hyperkalaemia: increased plasma potassium level

Hyperkeratosis: growth of keratinised tissue

Hypernatraemia: increased sodium blood level

Hypertension: increased blood pressure

Hyperthyroidism: increased activity of the thyroid gland

Hypoglycaemia: low blood glucose level

Hypokalaemia: low plasma potassium level

Hypothyroidism: decreased activity of the thyroid gland

Impetigo: skin infection

Iritis: inflammation of the iris

Ischaemic heart disease: diminished oxygen supply in the myocardial tissue cells

Ketonuria: excessive amounts of ketone bodies in the urine

Maculopapular eruptions: skin condition characterised by a rash consisting of distinct eruptions

Mania: psychiatric disorder characterised by agitation and elated mood

Multiple sclerosis: progressive degenerative disease presenting with disseminated demyelination of nerve fibres of the brain and spinal cord

Myalgia: muscle pain

Myasthenia gravis: a condition presenting with chronic fatigue and muscle weakness

Nappy rash: irritation in the napkin area, napkin dermatitis

Nephrotoxicity: toxic to the kidneys

Neural tube defects: congenital malformations of the skull and spinal cord resulting from failure of the neural tube to close during pregnancy

Nocturia: excessive urination at night

Oedema: accumulation of fluid in interstitial spaces

Onchomycosis: fungal nail infections

Osteoarthritis: arthritis associated with degenerative changes of the joints

Osteoporosis: loss of bone density

Otitis externa: inflammation or infection of the external ear

Otitis interna: labyrinthitis, inflammation or infection of the inner ear

Otitis media: inflammation or infection of the middle ear

Paget's disease: non-metabolic disease of the bones

Paraesthesia: numbness and tingling sensation

Parkinson's disease: progressive degenerative neurological disease characterised by tremors and muscle rigidity

Periodontitis: inflammation of the periodontium

Peripheral neuropathies: disorders of the peripheral nervous system

Polycystic ovary syndrome: endocrine disorder characterised by amenorrhoea, hirsutism and infertility

Porphyria: inherited disorders presenting with increased production of porphyrins in the bone marrow

Prostatic hyperplasia: enlargement of the prostate

Pseudomembranous colitis: diarrhoea occurring in patients who received antibacterial agents, caused by the resulting overgrowth of anaerobic bacteria in the gastrointestinal tract

Psoriasis: chronic skin condition presenting with red areas covered with dry, silvery scales

Rhinorrhoea: watery nasal discharge

Rosacea: chronic presentation of acne in adults characterised by dilation of the blood vessels of the face resulting in a flushed appearance

Seborrhoeic dermatitis: chronic inflammatory skin condition

Septicaemia: presence of pathogenic micro-organisms or their toxins in the bloodstream

Shingles: herpes zoster, infection due to the re-activation of the latent varicella zoster virus

Status epilepticus: occurrence of continuous seizures

Striae: scars in the skin

Tachycardia: heart rate more than 100 beats/min

Tardive dyskinesia: uncontrollable facial movements

Tinea corporis: ringworm infection

Tinea pedis: athlete's foot

Tinnitus: perception of sound such as buzzing, hissing or pulsating noises in the ears

Trigeminal neuralgia: pain and spasms along the trigeminal facial nerve

Typhoid fever: a bacterial infection caused by *Salmonella typhi*

Ulcerative colitis: chronic inflammatory disease affecting the large intestine and the rectum

Urticaria: a skin condition characterised by pruritus

Uterine fibroids: fibrous tissue growth in the uterus

Verrucas: viral skin infection, wart

Appendix C

Abbreviations and acronyms

5HT$_1$ agonist	serotonin receptor agonist type 1
5HT$_3$ antagonist	serotonin receptor antagonist type 3
ACE	angiotensin converting enzyme
AV node	atrioventricular node
BCG vaccine	Bacillus Calmette-Guerin vaccine
b.d.	twice daily
CAPD	continuous ambulatory peritoneal dialysis
CBC	complete blood count (full blood count)
CD	controlled drug
COPD	chronic obstructive pulmonary disease
COX-2 inhibitors	cyclo-oxygenase-2 inhibitors
CTZ	chemoreceptor trigger zone
FBC	full blood count
H$_2$-receptor	histamine type 2 receptor
HDL	high density lipoprotein
HMG CoA	3-hydroxy-3-methylglutaryl coenzyme A
INR	international normalised ratio
LDL	low density lipoprotein
m.	send, prepare
MAOI	monoamine oxidase inhibitor
NIDDM	non-insulin dependent diabetes mellitus
nocte	at night
NSAID	non-steroidal anti-inflammatory drug
o.d.	daily
o.m.	in the morning
o.n.	at night
OTC	over-the-counter preparation
p.c.	after food
PMH	past medical history
PND	paroxysmal nocturnal dyspnoea
p.r.n.	as required

q.d.s.	four times daily
RICE	rest, ice, compression and elevation
RIMA	reversible monoamine oxidase inhibitor type A
rINN	recommended International Non-proprietary Name
SPF	sun protection factor
SSRI	selective serotonin re-uptake inhibitor
TCA	tricyclic antidepressant
t.d.s.	three times daily
UVA	ultraviolet irradiation, long wavelengths
UVB	ultraviolet irradiation, medium wavelengths
w/v	weight in volume
w/w	weight in weight

Appendix D

Performance statistics

The tests were undertaken by a sample of final-year pharmacy students following a five-year course, which included the preregistration period. The percentage of students answering a question incorrectly is indicated for each test. Questions which were answered correctly by all students are not listed.

Test 1 (n = 36)

Question number	Students answering incorrectly (%)
1	3
2	22
3	28
4	6
6	25
7	25
8	22
10	11
11	28
13	14
14	3
15	3
16	31
17	3
18	14
19	8
21	14
22	3
23	22
25	3

Test 1 (n = 36) (continued)

Question number	Students answering incorrectly (%)
26	3
27	6
28	17
29	6
30	3
31	8
32	6
33	3
34	11
39	6
41	3
44	19
45	6
52	3
53	6
55	8
56	11
57	39
58	61
59	33
60	6
61	64
62	69
64	3
65	19
66	8
67	3
68	6
69	19
70	14
71	8
72	19

Test 1 (n = 36) (continued)

Question number	Students answering incorrectly (%)
73	44
74	22
75	19
76	8
77	8
78	11
79	11
80	17
81	3
82	11
83	25
84	28
85	31
86	72
87	8
88	8
89	3
90	14
91	3
92	39
93	11
94	17
95	11
96	31
97	44
98	3
99	22
100	11

Test 2 (n = 28)

Question number	Students answering incorrectly (%)
2	39
3	39
4	14
5	4
6	54
7	7
8	39
9	18
10	7
11	4
12	25
13	68
14	21
16	32
17	4
18	71
19	75
20	32
21	18
22	7
23	61
25	21
27	14
29	32
30	14
31	18
32	7
33	4
34	68
35	4
36	7
37	7

Test 2 (n = 28) (continued)

Question number	Students answering incorrectly (%)
38	32
43	39
44	18
53	82
54	82
55	11
56	82
57	43
58	11
59	4
60	36
61	14
62	11
63	18
64	18
65	18
66	7
67	36
68	14
69	36
70	89
71	46
72	46
73	21
74	39
75	39
76	14
77	7
78	21
79	11
80	32
81	4

Test 2 (n = 28) (continued)

Question number	Students answering incorrectly (%)
82	54
83	25
84	57
85	61
86	11
87	86
88	36
89	4
90	11
91	4
92	89
93	4
94	68
95	4
96	68
97	39
98	61
99	7
100	32

Test 3 (n = 32)

Question number	Students answering incorrectly (%)
1	6
2	3
4	34
5	3
6	6
7	3

Test 3 (n = 32) (continued)

Question number	Students answering incorrectly (%)
8	78
10	65
12	6
13	3
14	9
16	13
17	3
19	3
21	47
22	13
23	3
24	88
25	13
26	56
30	13
32	9
33	9
35	22
36	13
38	9
39	34
40	3
41	16
42	28
43	25
44	28
45	3
46	25
47	6
48	13
49	19
50	3

Test 3 (n = 32) (continued)

Question number	Students answering incorrectly (%)
51	13
52	41
53	9
54	28
55	19
56	22
57	31
58	6
59	47
60	6
61	6
62	3
63	41
64	13
65	38
66	19
67	28
70	44
71	28
72	31
73	3
74	9
75	75
76	9
77	6
78	9
79	56
80	25
81	53
82	9
83	3
84	25

Test 3 (n = 32) (continued)

Question number	Students answering incorrectly (%)
85	44
86	41
87	56
88	44
89	6
90	13
91	25
92	13
93	25
94	3
99	19
100	6

Test 4 (n = 36)

Question number	Students answering incorrectly (%)
1	8
2	17
3	69
4	11
6	17
7	17
8	3
9	61
10	14
11	8
14	6
15	17
16	6
17	3

Test 4 (n = 36) (continued)

Question number	Students answering incorrectly (%)
18	6
19	33
20	3
21	25
23	31
24	72
25	22
26	3
27	36
28	33
29	14
30	31
31	64
32	14
33	8
34	25
35	14
36	11
37	42
38	42
39	3
40	28
41	6
44	3
45	14
46	3
47	6
48	22
49	3
50	6
51	11
52	33

Test 4 (n = 36) (continued)

Question number	Students answering incorrectly (%)
53	6
54	19
55	58
56	64
57	8
58	8
59	97
60	47
61	3
62	47
63	39
64	47
65	92
66	14
67	19
68	47
69	6
70	3
71	22
73	22
74	6
75	78
76	25
77	83
78	17
80	78
81	11
82	50
83	6
84	61
87	19
88	3

Test 4 (n = 36) (continued)

Question number	Students answering incorrectly (%)
89	11
90	36
91	61
93	81
94	44
96	8
97	25
98	17
99	56
100	64

Test 5 (n = 28)

Question number	Students answering incorrectly (%)
1	7
2	50
3	29
4	43
5	43
6	43
7	18
8	4
9	50
10	14
11	50
12	11
13	21
14	7
15	14
16	4

Test 5 (n = 28) (continued)

Question number	Students answering incorrectly (%)
18	4
20	11
21	18
22	18
23	43
24	61
25	14
26	7
27	7
28	4
29	4
31	93
32	11
33	18
34	36
35	11
36	14
38	21
42	14
43	21
45	4
46	32
48	4
49	36
50	46
51	14
52	14
53	4
54	82
55	11
56	11
57	21

Test 5 (n = 28) (continued)

Question number	Students answering incorrectly (%)
58	61
59	18
60	18
61	7
62	82
63	32
64	29
65	50
66	46
67	7
68	21
69	25
70	11
71	18
72	50
73	4
74	21
75	79
76	75
77	86
78	43
79	96
80	57
81	68
82	14
83	7
84	89
85	36
86	36
88	7
89	86
90	25

Test 5 (n = **28**) (continued)

Question number	Students answering incorrectly (%)
91	11
92	29
93	25
94	11
95	11
96	14
97	11
98	4
99	61
100	14

Test 6 (n = 32)

Question number	Students answering incorrectly (%)
1	31
2	9
3	25
4	3
5	19
6	6
7	6
8	13
10	13
11	19
12	3
13	59
14	41
17	66
22	9
23	13

Test 6 (n = 32) (continued)

Question number	Students answering incorrectly (%)
25	13
27	3
29	3
30	16
32	16
33	38
34	4
36	3
37	22
38	38
42	78
43	10
44	22
45	22
46	16
47	10
49	31
54	3
55	25
56	3
57	13
61	3
62	59
63	63
64	66
65	10
66	3
67	6
68	28
69	44
71	41
72	13

Test 6 (**n** = **32**) (continued)

Question number	Students answering incorrectly (%)
73	31
74	44
75	9
76	44
77	19
78	31
79	22
80	50
81	3
82	25
83	25
85	3
86	69
87	31
88	22
89	28
90	53
91	66
92	31
93	28
94	3
95	3
96	59
97	9
98	38
99	31
100	13

Proprietary names index

Generic names index

Conditions index

Subject index